American Medical Association

Physicians dedicated to the health of America

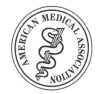

Assessing and Improving
Staffing and Organization

Prepared for
The American Medical Association
By Crystal S. Reeves

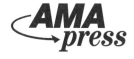

Assessing and Improving Staffing and Organization

Internet address: www.ama-assn.org

This book is for informational purposes only. It is not intended to constitute legal or financial advice. If legal, financial, or other professional advice is required, the services of a competent professional should be sought.

Additional copies of this book may be ordered by calling 800-621-8335. Secure on-line orders can be taken at www.ama-assn.org/catalog. Mention product number OP318500.

ISBN 1-57947-080-7
BP38:0092-00:10/00

THE COKER GROUP is a national provider of health care consultative and management services assisting physicians, hospitals, and health care systems to better position themselves to be successful in a reformed health care environment. THE COKER GROUP offers a broad spectrum of programs and services for its clients.

- Primary Care Physician Network Development
- Practice Valuations and Acquisition Negotiations
- Physician Employment and Compensation Contract Design
- Facilitation of Group Practice Development
- Physician Practice Management Services
- Management Services Organization (MSO) Development
- Market Share Management Program
- Newly Recruited Physician Services
- Educational Programs
- Evaluation and Consultant Services
- Personnel Productivity Programs
- *PRACTICE SUCCESS!*© and *PRACTICE SUCCESS!*© Series

For more information, contact

> The Coker Group
> 11660 Alpharetta Highway
> Building 700, Ste 710
> Roswell, GA 30076
> 678 832-2000
> www.cokergroup.com

ABOUT THE AUTHOR

Crystal S. Reeves, CPC, is a senior consultant in the Practice Services Division of The Coker Group, a national health care services firm specializing in physician development programs and other associated services. She has more than 20 years experience in health care and in medical practice management, working in a variety of settings, including internal medicine, endocrinology, neurosurgery, and neurology, and is certified by the American Academy of Professional Coders.

As a practice management consultant, Ms Reeves helps physicians and their staffs set up and strengthen business operations. Among the areas in which she has consulted are daily practice operations, billing and collection services, compliance issues, plan development, medical chart auditing, personnel management concerns, and start-up assistance for medical practices.

Ms Reeves is author of *The Renal Physicians Guide to Nephrology Practice* (Coker Consulting, LLC, and Renal Physicians Association, 1999) and *IPA Management: Legal and Compliance Guidelines* (McGraw-Hill, 1999). She is a frequent speaker at conferences and workshops on current topics in the health care field. She has also presented seminars nationwide on coding and reimbursement, documentation guidelines, managed care, and practice management.

ssessing and Improving Practice Staffing and Organization is one of a series of books written to provide assessment tools and systematic processes to enable internal examination of the strengths and weaknesses of business operations. With the right mechanisms in hand, the physician and practice manager will be able to take a fresh look at staffing, hiring, training, and assessment and to evaluate their effectiveness.

The purpose of this book is to provide step-by-step advice on developing an organization and building a staff that runs smoothly and efficiently. Developing a strong organization is essential to creating and maintaining ongoing revenue streams. Often, establishing and holding on to a thriving practice is less about the clinical astuteness of the physician and more about having the right people in place to maintain day-to-day operations. Included with this book is a diskette that contains many of the sample tables and forms in Microsoft Word® 6.0 for you to adapt, personalize, and modify for you and your practice.

This book and the others in the *Assessing and Improving Practice Operations*© Series are intended to offer concrete, practical information on topics sometimes considered the least important aspect of the profession of medicine: the business of running a medical practice. The long, hard years you dedicated to medical school and residency training were meant to make you an excellent physician, not an excellent businessperson. Caring for patients is and always will be your first priority. However, you cannot successfully run a medical practice without planning and without consideration of important business issues. While it takes a minimum of 10 years to become a physician, the day a practice opens is the day a physician becomes a small businessperson.

Your education probably did not include much information on medical office operations, personnel management, accounting, or business law. Yet, these business issues are more important than ever before, because the practice of medicine is far more complex than ever before. Good business management is essential to good medical practice. The physician who ignores basic business principles may soon face difficulties with suppliers, employees, the government, or patients.

Other pressures contribute to the need to seek greater efficiency. Most physicians find demands on their time increasing exponentially. There is a daily struggle to build a practice that will earn a steady income, to schedule regular working hours, to deliver quality care to patients, and to still have time for relaxation and family. Developing an efficient practice makes all of these attainable. The application of good business planning will enable you to spend more time on the things that are most important to you.

This book and the others in the *Assessing and Improving Practice Operations*© series are guides to medical practice management for both the new physician and the established physician. They are not intended to provide solutions to every challenge that may arise. Their goal is to acquaint you with essential business principles and tools, as well as with some new approaches to managing your practice. The information they provide can be supplemented with information you gather from your colleagues and advisors. You will then be in a position to explore those ideas that promise to achieve the best results for your particular situation.

By providing the information in this book and others, the American Medical Association (AMA) is not endorsing any one management philosophy or method of delivering health care services. No single approach will meet the objectives of all physicians. Physicians and their staffs have to decide for themselves the best way to manage their individual practices. Finally, this book does not enunciate AMA policy. The annual *Policy Compendium* of the AMA sets forth our positions on such issues as contracting, medical ethics, managed care, and practice management.

We hope that this publication will be useful to you.

The American Medical Association

CONTENTS

CONTENTS

LIST OF FIGURES, FORMS, AND TABLES

Figures

Forms

Tables

LIST OF FIGURES, FORMS, AND TABLES

CHAPTER 1

Defining the Organization's Vision and Mission

The partners of Good Health Family Clinic had been sitting around the conference table for 3 hours trying to figure out what went wrong. Just a year ago, they had held their annual planning session at this same hotel. The physicians had left the meeting feeling that they had accomplished a lot. They had reviewed the year's finances, set goals for making more money, and agreed that the coming year would be one of the best. They knew that managed care had cut into their profits considerably and that they had to find ways to make up that loss. During the planning session, they had looked for ways to cut costs, and each physician outlined his plans for bringing more money into the practice.

However, contrary to their expectations, profits decreased even more. The clinic was experiencing significant staff turnover and a decline in patient satisfaction. There was a lot of blame-placing and finger-pointing—and of course there was the whole managed care issue.

Now they were reflecting on that meeting a year ago to find out what they could do this year to make things turn out differently.

LESSONS LEARNED

Drs Benz, Daniel, and Stock were just beginning to see that it takes more to keep a successful business going than cutting costs, watching the bottom line, and finding new ways to make money. All of these actions are important, but it takes more than money to energize an organization and keep it moving forward. The decisions the physicians made during their annual planning session were all money-driven reactions to the managed care market. Instead of establishing clear goals for the clinic, the physicians set their own goals and behaved as if they were in private practices. The staff turnover and decline in patient satisfaction were additional indicators that this practice was in trouble.

What could have helped Good Health Family Clinic? One of the most important things the physicians could have done at their annual planning meeting would have been to discuss where they saw their practice in 5 years. What did they value in their lives? What did they stand for as a group? What did they envision their practice being?

At least one person in the group should have had a vision about where health care was going and should have been able to define a course of action that would bring changes to the practice. Ideally, that leader would be someone who was not only able to assume risk, but was also able to build a cohesive team that would support management's goals.

In the first planning retreat, each physician listed individual goals for the practice, but they failed to bring all the individual goals and preferences into one big picture. If they had done so, they may have seen that pursuing many different goals and dreams (while also trying to cut expenses) would overtax a practice that was already suffering from reduced revenues.

The first step any organization should take is to determine its goals. To facilitate the task of determining which goals to pursue, begin by establishing a mission statement.

WHAT IS A MISSION STATEMENT?

A mission statement identifies the purpose of an organization. It defines who you are, how you treat your employees, how you relate to your patients, and how departments interact with each other. The mission statement is the DNA of the organization.

It is important to understand the real purpose of such a statement and what the statement should say about the organization. The mission statement should be an inspiring statement, not only to physicians and top managers, but also to rank-and-file staff members. It should provide guidance to help people respond to daily events and daily operational problems. It should serve as a touchstone to evaluate the direction the practice is going and the decisions that are being made. A good mission statement should also be a reminder of why the practice exists. From this foundation, the mission statement can be translated into a strategic plan, and it will also determine how the practice regards and treats its employees.

TOOLS FOR DEFINING YOUR MISSION

If you work for an organization that already has a mission statement (for example, a hospital or physician practice management organization), you may think this part has already been done for you. However, you may want to review that mission statement and ask whether the statement really belongs to you, if it is your touchstone for running your practice. If it is not, can you expand on it to make it your own? Would your office or department have a more cohesive feeling if you worked on establishing a mission statement that complemented the existing one?

Depending on your answers, you may want to consider developing a statement for your office or department that supports and enhances the broader mission statement. On the other hand, if you have had your mission statement for several years, you may want to review it and ask:

1. Is this mission statement still relevant to today's needs?
2. Is our practice for the most part unchanged since the statement was developed?
3. Is this statement a living part of the current organization's culture?

If you answered no to two or all three of these questions, you may want to consider updating the existing mission statement or starting all over with a new mission for a new office.

STEPS FOR CREATING A MISSION STATEMENT

How do you go about developing a mission statement for your practice and stating that mission so that it unifies and inspires people? The steps described following will help you develop a statement that your organization can be proud of and use for years to come.

Step 1: Assembling the Vision Team

The vision team should consist of representatives from every department of the organization. The more people who have input into the development of the mission, the greater the ultimate buy-in from everyone. Post a notice inviting everyone who is interested to be part of the team. (See **Figure 1-1.**) Asking for volunteers rather than designating representatives from each department will promote the acceptance of the statement once completed.

The notice outlines the benefit of participation. It should also either list a name for participants to contact or the time and place of the meeting.

You may want to generate interest by getting the names of interested parties, and post the meeting notice later. Those who were not prompted to call after reading the first notice may decide to attend the meeting. When the list is finalized, announce the members of the vision team. See **Form 1-1.**

FIGURE 1-1. VISION TEAM NOTICE

BE PART OF OUR VISION TEAM

We are looking for energetic, enthusiastic people to be part of the team that develops our new mission and values statement. This statement will define who we are as a practice and formalize the values, beliefs, and ethical standards of our organization.

As a member of the Vision Team, you will be part of the most important aspect of our organization—defining who we are and for what we stand.

For more information contact:

FORM 1-1. VISION TEAM MEMBERS

Name	Job Title	Department	Extension

The leader of the vision team plays a crucial role not only in developing the mission statement but also in the success of the statement in changing the behavior of the organization. The leader serves as a psychological focal point in the mission and strategic planning process.

Step 2: Electing the Leader

The leader who is selected should be

- Visioning. This individual can create a realistic picture of the future and convey that picture to other team members and to the organization as a whole.
- Energizing. A good vision leader generates excitement and energy for the entire team. The enthusiasm is contagious, and other vision team members become more animated and committed to the mission as a result of this leadership.
- Enabling. This person helps others perform. The entire team will play better as a result of this person's leadership ability.

Form 1-2 shows a grid that assists in selecting a good team leader.

FORM 1-2. TEAM LEADER SELECTION GRID

Quality	Candidate 1	Candidate 2	Candidate 3	Candidate 4
Will invest the necessary time in the project				
Has a reputation for getting things done				
Will address this endeavor in a timely fashion				
Demonstrates vision in his or her everyday work style				
Energizes others in a working group				
Can stimulate others to better performance				

Vision Team Leader Name _____

Step 3: Vision Team Meeting

Once the team is formed and the leader selected, the next step is to meet to begin the design. The purpose of the first session is to introduce basic education pertaining to developing a mission statement, describing what you are looking for, outlining what the result will be used for, and establishing what is expected of team members. **Table 1-1** is a sample meeting agenda.

TABLE 1-1. SAMPLE MEETING AGENDA

Purpose:
To define who we are as a business by developing a mission statement.

Items for Discussion:

I. What is the objective of a mission statement?
The purpose of a mission statement is to

- Define the business

- Define what we want the practice to be like in a few years

- Identify the changes occurring in medicine that affect the way we will practice

- Determine what we must do to ensure that the practice will have the characteristics we desire

The mission statement should also state objectives that can be measured, and that are relevant to all stakeholders.

II. What are the characteristics of a good mission statement?
A good mission statement can accomplish the following:

- Change the practice's behavior

- Excite and inspire

- State what the practice chooses to do in order to thrive, not state what the practice should do to survive

One of the most common mistakes in formulating a mission statement is to state the obvious. For example, "To provide the best quality patient care and still make a profit," states a goal with which few people would disagree. Yet, can you imagine this statement motivating employees? The mission statement should challenge people and promote innovation. For example, it could be worded as follows:

Our company philosophy is

- to serve our customers with a sense of competitive urgency,
- to be ethical in dealing with our customers and employees,
- to have the courage to face facts and to follow the facts even into unfamiliar and unexplored territory,
- to be consistent in quality and in performance, and
- to pursue our business and our jobs with enthusiasm.

This statement is inspirational. It has lofty, yet attainable, goals. It challenges employees to reach for the stars. This is the kind of statement to create. So, how do you go about doing so? Involve all members of the vision team through the following process.

First, define the aspirations of the organization. Give participants pads of Post-it® notes, and ask them to write their answers to the following questions. These are their aspiration statements.

A year from now

1. What will our patients say about us?
2. What will our competitors say about us?
3. What will our employees say about us?
4. What standards of excellence will we have achieved?
5. What will our reputation be?
6. Where will we be in the marketplace?

Next, compile the aspiration statements for each category. Place large sheets of paper on the wall with one question written on each sheet. As the members complete their answers, they can stick the Post-it® notes under the appropriate questions.

Then, identify the guiding principles of the organization. Have the team members write their responses to the following questions regarding guiding principles of the organization:

1. How will we treat our patients?
2. How will we treat employees?
3. How will we conduct our business?
4. How will we treat other physicians?
5. How will we treat our vendors, suppliers, and other people with whom we do business?
6. How will we treat our community?
7. How will we treat our environment?

Next, compile the guiding principles. Place seven large sheets of paper on the wall corresponding to the seven categories of guiding principles. Have participants place their notes on the appropriate sheet.

Now, divide the group into six subgroups, each of which will work on developing one aspiration category into one consensus statement and three or four guiding principles. This will take approximately 20 to 30 minutes. When the aspirations are finalized, have each group make its presentation, allowing the team to ask questions and discuss the aspirations.

Once the group has agreed on the aspirations, it is now time to consolidate them into a single statement. This may be one sentence or a paragraph or two. It should respond to all six questions posed, but it does not have to correlate one-on-one to each question.

Then, put the mission statement to the test. (See **Table 1-2.**) Finalize the statement by asking the following questions.

- Does this statement reflect what we want this practice to be like in a few years?
- Will this statement serve us through the changes that are occurring in medicine, in our community, our patients, and our competition?
- What will we have to begin to do now in order to ensure that our practice will have these characteristics?
- Most importantly, does this statement challenge us to a higher goal?

If the vision team feels that the developed statement meets the needs of the organization, it is ready to be presented. If, however, there is doubt, lack of enthusiasm, or failure to energize, the team may want to meet one more time to refine, revise, or completely redefine the mission statement.

If the mission is well developed, it will lead the organization for years to come. It should serve as an inspiration for achievement, promote interaction among all employees, and provide the springboard to a good strategic plan.

A mission statement coupled with a well-designed strategic plan can identify major activities that are required to attain the vision of the company. And vision will take the organization out of the past and commit it to the future.

TABLE 1-2. SELF-TEST FOR SUCCESSFUL MISSION AND VISION

Yes	No	
❏	❏	We have defined in finite terms where we want to be in 5 years.
❏	❏	We have a leader to focus our attention on the future.
❏	❏	We have involved people from all departments and staff levels in the development of our mission.
❏	❏	Our mission statement defines how we will treat our patients, our employees, and each other.
❏	❏	The mission statement inspires us to reach for a higher goal.

MISTAKES TO AVOID

- Failing to develop any kind of mission statement
- Developing a mission statement quickly so as to move on with a strategic plan
- Developing a mission statement that does not motivate nonmanagerial employees
- Trying to develop a mission statement without a shared vision

CHAPTER 2

Identifying the Culture

Western Internal Medicine Associates is made up of four physicians—Dr Albert plus three partners he has taken in over the years. Dr Albert has been in practice since the mid-1960s. The practice has been in its current location for more than 25 years. Dr Albert has always been the managing partner, which means there is no office manager or practice manager. Dr Albert fills that role in addition to performing his medical responsibilities.

Things have changed at the practice over the years—but minimally and slowly. Dr Albert still keeps track of employee time in his ledger book and writes the paychecks by hand. An employee who wants time off writes him a note and places it on his desk. Dr Albert approves all purchases and makes all decisions about the direction of the practice. He does not like midlevel providers and in fact will not permit another physician's midlevel provider to see his patients in the hospital. He also resents being referred to as a "provider" when he is in fact a "physician."

His office reflects the style of the 1960s—his charts have no fasteners, and the office notes look much as they did when he first started practicing. Little change has occurred in this practice. Yet, the employees are used to his ways and the practice experiences little turnover.

Dan Internal Medicine is quite different from Western Internal Medicine Associates. Dr Dan is a new physician just starting an internal medicine practice. He wants his practice to be state of the art in every way, and he invested considerable sums in order to buy cutting-edge equipment and make his office esthetically pleasing to his patients. He searched for an electronic medical records package that would allow him to have a paperless office. His two employees call him by his first name, and he treats them to lunch frequently.

Within 6 months of opening his doors, Dr Dan added a physician's assistant so that he could grow his practice. He believes in sufficient time off to relax and regroup, and he provides his employees with generous time-off packages. Decisions are group decisions, although Janice, the office manager, may at times override the group decision. This practice is always looking for ways to improve.

These examples reflect actual internal medicine practices with very different cultures. What do you think would happen if an employee from Dr Dan's practice went to work at Western Internal Medicine Associates? What do you think would happen if an employee from Western Internal Medicine Associates went to work at Dan Internal Medicine? Do you think they would feel comfortable in their new environment? Would they be happier or less happy in their new office? Do you think they would stay with the new job?

LESSONS LEARNED

Although both of these practices are internal medicine practices operating in the western portion of the United States, they are vastly different in their management styles and culture. If you looked into how each practice treats its employees and its patients, and what character traits and talents are valued at each practice, you would probably find that the practices differed in many ways besides management style.

All the traits, habits, beliefs, and idiosyncrasies of an organization are known as its culture—an intangible software of the mind that is part of the identity of people and their organizations. Culture, in its simplest form, is how you do things in the organization. It plays a crucial role in employee selection, training, motivation, and retention. It influences how you make decisions and determines who will fit in, feel comfortable, and become an effective member of your team, and who will probably seek employment elsewhere. Therefore, to build a cohesive team to help reach your vision, it is important to define the culture of your organization. Then you need to hire employees who will support that culture.

By defining and understanding the culture of your practice, you will be able to

- provide a clear profile of the kind of employee you want to hire,
- draw a clear picture of what skills to test,
- identify good questions to ask during an interview,
- determine on what to focus during orientation,
- establish and develop training programs that support the culture, and
- mentor employees, coach them for success, and build a winning team.

EXAMINING THE CULTURE

Regardless of the product it delivers, every company faces the same problems and challenges, including authority relationships, conflict, growth and expansion issues, and competition for market share. How companies solve these problems differs. The more clearly you can identify the method your organization uses to meet these problems, the better you will be able to manage.

Culture is really an extension of the mission statement. It defines who you are as a company and clarifies your norms. It governs how people relate to one another, the level of openness of the communication, and how decisions are made. New employees will quickly learn what it takes to succeed in your organization by observing the culture.

However, some cultures are hard to define, especially if employees have been working in an organization for a long time. One way to assess an organization's culture is to look at **Figure 2-1,** which identifies three equal sides to cultural dimensions: tasks, orientation, and communication style.

FIGURE 2-1. DIMENSIONS IN CULTURAL MANAGEMENT

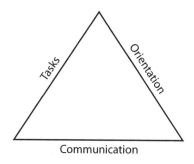

How do you approach tasks in your organization? Some organizations approach tasks in a very structured way with written policies and standard operating procedures. Others provide fewer formal task directives or may have no written guidelines at all.

Side 1: Tasks

Does the organization approach work by focusing on the task or by looking at the people involved in the task (process or people)? For example, one health care system met the challenge of employee turnover by developing a charge-capturing system that was so refined it involved no thought on the part of the person entering the data. Anyone who sat in the poster's seat could enter the data with minimal training. The process was

Side 2: Orientation

all that mattered in that case. The people were interchangeable and contributed very little to accomplishing the task.

Side 3: Communication Style

How do your employees communicate with each other and with supervisors? Is communication primarily by memos and electronic messaging, or is it done informally in the break room, by handwritten notes on the bulletin board, or through "oh, by the ways" shouted down the halls?

By measuring these three dimensions of cultural management, we begin to get an idea of how our organization operates. You will need to begin the culture identification process by answering some questions about your organization, starting with organization tasks.

TOOLS FOR DEFINING THE CULTURE

Complete the following exercise to define the culture of your practice.

Dimension 1: Tasks

1. How does your organization approach tasks?
2. Are well-defined process descriptions followed religiously for each task that is completed?
3. Do you give employees jobs to do and allow them to complete the jobs their own way?
4. Do you have standard protocols and structured tasks for the clinical side of your practice, but adopt a more casual approach to check-in, appointment scheduling, and sending out bills?
5. Do you have well-defined task descriptions but tend to ignore them when things get busy?
6. Do all departments approach tasks the same way?
7. Is the practice content with the way tasks are approached, or do the physicians and/or employees long for it to be different?
8. How do they want?
9. Do they recognize the advantages and disadvantages of both methods?
10. Have you had discussions regarding the accepted approach to tasks?

Dimension 2: Orientation

The next measurable dimension is orientation.

1. Is your culture task-oriented or people-oriented? Most practices are people-oriented cultures for their customers.

2. How does it work internally? Is the manager inclined to whiz in, sort things out, get out, and do the next job? Or is the manager more apt to establish and build a relationship before looking at the problem?

3. What does your organization value—teamwork or bottom-line results? Getting to work or working together?

4. Do you have regular staff meetings to sort things out and discuss issues?

5. Does everyone—including physicians—attend them?

6. Are people given time to talk through a work-related problem so that they can develop a better way of doing things?

7. Are new employees allowed to get their bearing and become comfortable in the job, or are they expected to hit the ground running?

8. Are your most valued employees inclined to be task-oriented or people-oriented?

Finally, we come to the communication style of the practice.

Dimension 3: Communication

1. Is communication factual or expressive? Naturally, medical records and bills are factual, but how do workers communicate with each other? Do you have formal lines of communication that follow your organization chart, or do you have an open-door policy starting with physicians and moving on through the ranks? Do you send out memos when you want to get a point across or scrawl a note on a blackboard next to the nurses station? Are people open to popping their heads in the door and relaying a message, or are communications formalized from one person to the other? Is humor in good taste common, or do people raise their eyebrows at an attempt at levity? Communication tells a lot about your organization.

2. Does your organization make extensive use of memos and written communication?

3. If you wanted to tell the physicians something about a staffing problem, how would you do it?

4. If new employees wanted to talk with you, would you (a) ask them to write you a note requesting an appointment, (b) tell them you are not their immediate supervisor and to go through the ranks, or (c) suggest you have lunch together to talk?

5. Does your office communication system rely heavily on (a) schmoozing around the coffeepot, (b) intraoffice voice mail, (c) notes left on the person's desk, or (d) regularly scheduled meetings?

Once you have thought about these questions, ask other members of your organization to answer the same questions so that you have several people's opinions on how the organization works. If you find several people agreeing with you on the dimensions of tasks, orientation, and communication, you can then move on to assessing your ambiguity tolerance. If you find that there are differing answers to these questions, additional investigation is recommended. Although you may think you have an open-door policy, for example, others may perceive management as being very closed to accepting questions from employees. At the same time, although management believes it is sending out ample memos on subjects, those who "need to know" may believe they are always left out. Roundtable discussion and meetings will help discover why there are these different perceptions and facilitate future communication.

AMBIGUITY TOLERANCE TEST

The next measure of an organization's culture is in its flexibility in leaving things open. For example, cultures that have low tolerance for ambiguity tend to be highly structured and well-organized, have clear agendas for meetings and follow those agendas, have a time consciousness, and work through issues with a step-by-step approach.

An organization that has a high tolerance for ambiguity may believe that planning is not that important, but that it is important for the goal to be achieved regardless of the method. Employees may be encouraged to "go with the flow" and change direction easily. Such an organization does not bother drawing up agendas.

Health care organizations tend to be more highly structured. Among practices themselves, however, there is a high degree of diversity in the ambiguity tolerance factor. You need to be aware of the difference in health care relative to other businesses and to the wide variety of cultures within the field. For example, say that you hire a network administrator who has been accustomed to working in an environment with little structure. In his last position, he could do his work at his discretion, as long as the work got done. Your expectations are different, however. Both you and the new administrator might find yourselves frustrated if you expect him to be at work promptly at 8 o'clock each morning, to document everything he does in the course of work, and to attend numerous highly structured meetings. On the other hand, a nurse who is used to working in a highly structured hospital environment may find your office culture to be too undefined or lacking professionalism.

The point is that there is no right or wrong organizational culture. Obviously, the culture that focuses on the people and builds and develops a strong staff is a more desirable place to work. However, when it comes to tasks, communication, orientation, and ambiguity tolerance, it is advisable to know your own culture before you hire people to work in it.

CULTURAL INVENTORY

The following questions will help you develop an inventory of your organization.

1. Does your organization value risk-taking?
2. What happens when an employee challenges the status quo?
3. Do you develop and support leaders from within?
4. Do your departments work together as a team, or individually?
5. Are there boundaries and barriers to teamwork (eg, nursing staff versus lab; front desk versus nursing staff)?
6. Do you participate actively in benchmarking?
7. Do you want to be cutting-edge leaders in the field?
8. What authority do staff members have?
9. What mistakes should never be made?
10. What rate of failure is acceptable?
11. How do physicians treat staff members?
12. Are the physicians paternalistic in their approach to staff members, or do they take a team approach?
13. Do staff members feel a kinship with each other?
14. Do you socialize frequently outside the office, or do you have work relationships only?
15. Are newcomers readily accepted?
16. Do you have so many newcomers that no one pays attention to them until they've been there a while?
17. What is valued in your organization? Exceptional brilliance? The person who brings in the most money? The person who works well with others? The person who puts in extra time on nights and weekends? The person who has the best relationship with patients? The person who has the most education?
18. Do you have regular formal meetings or mini catch-ups?
19. Do people greet each other every day when first arriving at the office?
20. Are you a laid-back group or more inclined to be workaholics?

21. Do you often hear, "We've always done it that way" or "We tried that, and it didn't work"?

22. Do you have a way of trying new ideas and suggestions?

23. Do patients really come first?

24. If there was a patient on the telephone who needed assistance and a physician who needed help, who would be considered more important?

24. Do people regularly receive positive feedback for a job well done?

Once you and other staff members have answered these questions, you will have a clearer picture of the culture of your organization. You will know if you are a culture of innovation, risk-taking, and continuous improvement, or a more reserved structured entity that focuses on tasks and procedures.

MISTAKES TO AVOID

- Believing that only one culture is acceptable
- Not seeing your organization clearly
- Ignoring culture when hiring new employees
- Using culture as an excuse for not changing

CHAPTER 3

Determining the Best Structure

In 1969, when Dr Radcliff finished his residency and was ready to begin practicing medicine, he started his own practice. His wife, Sandra, was his receptionist and bookkeeper, and he hired a nurse to assist him. In 1972, he hired another physician, Dr Powers, to share the workload and help him build the practice. He also hired a nurse to work with Dr Powers. Sandra was still able to handle the workload at the front desk.

As Dr Powers developed his practice, the workload increased to the extent that the practice hired another person to assist Sandra in the front office. When they hired a third doctor, they had to hire another part-time receptionist, and Sandra decided to quit work. The doctors decided that Liz, who was Sandra's assistant, would become the office manager.

The nurses who had been with the doctors a long time did not want to report to an office manager when they had been reporting directly to the doctors. The newly hired employees, a full-time transcriptionist and a part-time medical records specialist, were content with reporting to the new office manager. So the doctors decided that the nurses would report directly to them, and the front office administrative staff would report to the office manager.

As new physicians were introduced into the practice and staff was hired to support them, the structure of the organization became more fragmented. The physicians continued to operate as a partnership, with all partners having an equal say in all of the decisions. Therefore, the decision-making process required the office manager to gain consensus from five, six, or seven partners before taking action. Little got accomplished. The once highly successful practice began experiencing employee turnover, physician discontent, mounting accounts receivables, and financial stress. For those who had witnessed the growth and prosperity of the practice, the question was, "What went wrong?"

LESSONS LEARNED

This practice is not unlike many others that either never really finalized the organizational structure or failed to make changes to the structure as the practice grew and evolved. Often, newly formed or small health care organizations do not see the need to have formalized organizational structures. Many practices start out with everyone reporting to the physician, and they never address changes that need to be made. In multiphysician practices, it is sometimes politically advantageous to neglect a formal structure so as to offend no one.

However, many large organizations have found that they can reduce turnover if employees have clear definitions of where they fit in. For example, the turnover rate at Index Systems, a multimillion-dollar programming firm, once jumped from 15% to greater than 30%. The problem was traced to the fact that the company was not overly concerned with titles, lines of authority, or formal structure. Employees were confused about lines of authority and structure. When structure was implemented, the number of employees doubled from 100 to 200, sales increased 40% annually, and the turnover rate dropped from 30% to 15%.[1]

In many cases, office staff members move up through the ranks to occupy the chair of office manager by default. It may become evident that the staff member who became manager by default is not the best person for the job. But rather than face the consequences of removing him or her, the physician develops a job description around that person. The resulting circumventing organization chart looks something like the one in **Figure 3-1.**

FIGURE 3-1. CIRCUMVENTING ORGANIZATION CHART

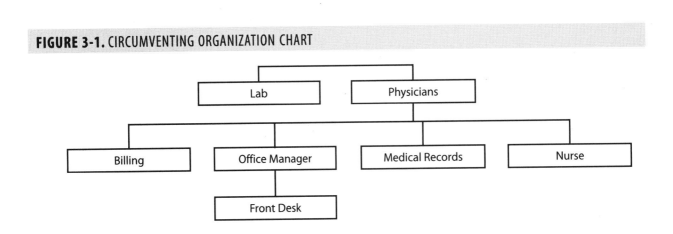

A similar version of this organizational structure develops when practices grow and change but fail to address the formal structure and reporting methods in the practice. The result looks similar to the appendage organizational structure as seen in **Figure 3-2.**

Often, practices that do have some built-in structure fail to update their organization charts as jobs and circumstances change. Many physicians do not like the formality of designing an organizational structure because their leadership and decision-making authorities are vague. Nevertheless, organizational structure is a vital part of determining and identifying the nature of a practice. Structure defines lines of accountability and outlines how people and departments relate to each other. Structure exists to accomplish the vision of the organization. It is a vital part of what a practice is.

In designing organization structures, health care managers are inclined to think in one of two ways. They may believe that the health care industry is so distinct and unique that none of the organizational structures can actually serve the medical practice's needs. On the other hand they feel that they need organizational structure and pattern the health care organization after manufacturing, retail, or commercial businesses. To determine what organizational structures to use for your organization, look at the organizational chart itself, how the departments and divisions are lined up and interact, and the policies and procedures that govern that structure.

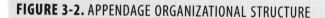

FIGURE 3-2. APPENDAGE ORGANIZATIONAL STRUCTURE

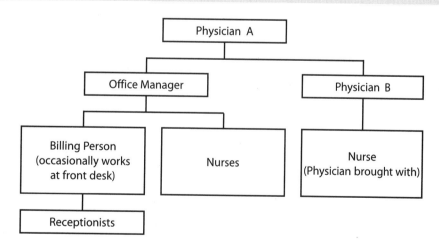

THE ORGANIZATIONAL CHART

In the simplest organizational chart, all employees report to one physician. Many smaller practices start with a simple organizational structure similar to the one in **Figure 3-3.** In this structure, all the upward and downward communication takes place to and from the physician. The advantage of this structure is that it can provide the physician with a lot of information about the daily operations of the practice. The lines are simple and direct. However, the disadvantage is that the physician is handling all staff problems and making sure that all the contributions fit together to ensure the smooth running of the practice.

Therefore, as practices grow and the number of employees increases, most physicians find this organizational structure too time-consuming. They usually establish an office manager position that will act as a buffer between the physician and the staff members. The structure's additional layer of people might look something like **Figure 3-4.** In this structure, effective communication is essential between physician and office manager and between office manager and staff. It is necessary to hold regular meetings to apprise the physician of what is occurring in the office. This structure removes the physician from the daily operations, which can be a benefit or a detriment. The success of the practice is now partly vested in another person. How that person supports the physician's vision, relates to staff, and carries communication back to the physician and staff will have a great effect on the success—or failure—of the organization.

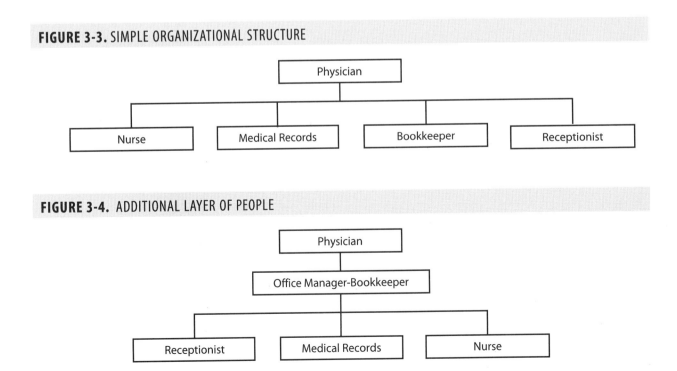

FIGURE 3-3. SIMPLE ORGANIZATIONAL STRUCTURE

FIGURE 3-4. ADDITIONAL LAYER OF PEOPLE

Often, the bookkeeper or the front office worker is named office manager. In many cases, this individual is fully capable of assuming the additional responsibilities. In some cases, he or she is not. Typically, he or she was not hired for his or her management skills and seldom has prior management experience. The individual may work well in a small office environment and may grow into the expanded job as he or she gains experience and additional training. However, some individuals are not meant to be managers, and instead of pulling the office together, their lack of management skills can induce staff turnover and declining morale.

It is important to remember that a great employee is not necessarily management material. Transitioning from a structure where the physician is manager to a practice under the direction of an office manager calls for as much care in selecting the office manager as if you were selecting a chief executive officer for a Fortune 500 company. With the right manager, you may someday be as successful as a Fortune 500 company.

Often, as practices grow and physicians incorporate or form large partnerships, having a physician serve as director may no longer be workable. There may be many physicians in positions of authority. When that happens, the practice may form an executive committee, and the new organizational structure may look like the one in **Figure 3-5.** All owners are part of the committee, and the committee directs the workings of the practice. The advantage of this type of structure is that no physician has more decision-making authority than the others. The directors, often with the office manager, meet as a group to make decisions. The office manager then runs the practice based on those decisions. To avoid having to call a meeting each time a decision needs physician input, the physicians are assigned management areas. Usually they are given guidelines about the types of decision and dollar amounts they can authorize without going back to the board for discussion. The disadvantage of this type of structure is that the physicians are even farther removed from the daily operations of

FIGURE 3-5. ORGANIZATIONAL STRUCTURE WITH EXECUTIVE COMMITTEE

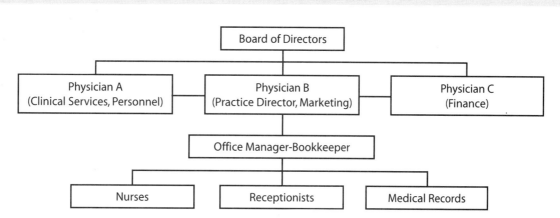

the practice. Depending on the size of the practice, the structure can also place a great deal of responsibility on the office manager.

As practices grow, the model shown in **Figure 3-6** may prove to be more advantageous. The office manager (or practice manager) oversees the big picture, while responsibilities for staffing are divided among department supervisors. This structure is beginning to resemble that of larger corporations. It has departments, department supervisors, and layers of management. The advantage is that no one person has an overload of direct reports. As practices grow, there is no efficient method for managing the staff members without dividing authority among several people.

The disadvantage, however, is that as more layers are added, the physicians are farther removed from the daily operations, and they are apt to be unaware of the thinking of the rank-and-file. As the structure grows, even the office manager (or practice manager, as the position evolves) is removed from the daily operations of the practice. The structure begins to resemble a bureaucracy, and decision-making may be slowed and encumbered. The structure shown in **Figure 3-7,** which is usually seen in hospital-owned practices or departments, takes physicians completely out of the management process.

FIGURE 3-6. MODEL FOR LARGER PRACTICES

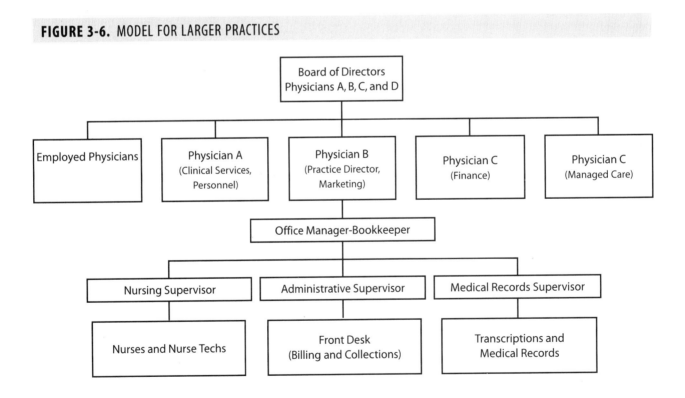

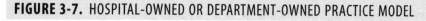

FIGURE 3-7. HOSPITAL-OWNED OR DEPARTMENT-OWNED PRACTICE MODEL

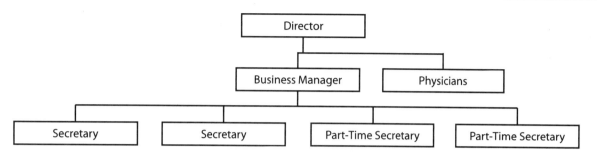

One disadvantage of organizational structures is that they often exist only on paper and have little effect on the practice. "Sure, we have an organizational structure, but no one follows it," may be the sentiment of the staff. Employees who are supposed to be reporting to a supervisor may actually report to the office manager, or staff members may ignore the lines of communication. The purpose of a good organizational structure is to facilitate communication. If the structure is not being implemented, it is not promoting communication. If it is actually hindering contact and interaction, then the structure needs to be reviewed.

After studying many types of organizations and many types of organizational structures, Henry Mintzberg determined that there are alternate paths to success. In fact, "getting it all together proved more important than any one best way."[2]

HOW DEPARTMENTS AND DIVISIONS LINE UP AND INTERACT

When determining the structure of your organization, determine whether each job is a line function or a staff function. Line functions do the work (eg, radiology, nursing, and laboratory); staff functions support the work (eg, personnel and payroll).

Health care organizations need people in both line functions and the staff functions. However, this is often where communications break down or avenues of communications are lost. For instance, a billing person (staff function) may not feel comfortable approaching a physician (line function) about how things are marked on a superbill. Likewise, an employee in the office medical records department (staff function) may not want a receptionist (line function) giving directions on chart/record management. An organization chart with clearly drawn lines of communication will help prevent misunderstandings and avoid inadequate interaction between functions.

POLICIES AND PROCEDURES THAT GOVERN

Defining the organization on paper is the first step in determining the structure of an organization. The second step is to look at how the boxes on the organization chart relate, interact, and communicate. In short, you need to look at how to do the things you do.

Organizations generally fall in between the two systems of organization that are outlined in **Table 3-1.** At one end is the job organization system. This system involves highly repetitive jobs. Usually it has a highly detailed approach to management, and the whole system can be controlled fairly closely. In a job organization system, the workers show up, do the job, and work to get paid.

On the other end of the scale is the cooperative motivation system. This system evolved in work environments where variable work dominates. In this system, management is less refined or defined. Jobs are not readily definable, and it is impossible to maintain specific controls over an activity. In a cooperative motivation system, the work depends on motivation and working together with other individuals.

The basic structure of a professional organization is usually somewhat bureaucratic without being centralized. Typically, the work is complex and carried out by controlled professionals. The work of those professionals can be perfected through standard operating programs. The professional organizational structure is common in universities, general hospitals, accounting firms, and physicians' offices. All rely on the skills and knowledge of their professional employees. Customarily, professionals are given control over their own work, and they usually work independently as colleagues. In fact, many professionals work more closely with their clients (patients) than they do with their coworkers.

TABLE 3-1. ORGANIZATION SCALES

JOB ORGANIZATION SYSTEMS	COOPERATIVE MOTIVATION SYSTEMS
• Repetitive movement	• Variable work
• High degree of organization	• Management is less refined
• High control of environment	• Jobs not readily defined in small details
• Depends on economic motives	• Less opportunity for close control
• Can define jobs in great detail	• Job depends on the individual

DETERMINING YOUR ORGANIZATION'S STRUCTURE

Where does your organization sit on the scale of organizations? Start by establishing the line functions of your practice. Write the name of each line function (eg, laboratory, radiology, physicians, nursing) on a self-adhesive note. Place the notes on a flat surface. Then write the staff functions (eg, billing, front desk, bookkeeping) on a different color note, and place them on the surface.

Determine to whom each of these functions directly reports. (Whom do they call when they cannot come to work?) Write the titles of the supervisors on notes, and place them above each function. Continue this process until you have reached the line where the function reports to no one, at which point you will be finished.

Next, determine how the departments interact.

- Is there anyone who reports to two or more people?
- Are there any supervisory lines that look out of place?
- How do people on the first line relate to all the people on the second line?
- How do people on second line relate to people on the third line?
- How do managers communicate and interact with each other?
- Are there any barriers to communication?
- How long does it take a suggestion to make its way up for approval?

Once you are satisfied the departments can communicate with each other effectively, consider the standard operating policies in each department.

- Are the policies designed to promote the best patient care?
- Are policies necessary to protect patient confidentiality?
- Do policies prevent errors?
- Do policies promote better department interactions?
- Are there policies that hinder performance?
- Are there written policies that hinder work flow for no known reason?

ASSESSING HOW WELL YOUR CURRENT ORGANIZATION IS DEFINED

The following checklist will help you assess how well your current organization is defined.

- Do you have an established organization chart?
- Is it on paper?
- Or is it an unwritten part of the culture?
- Are lines of communication clear to all workers?
- Have there been any disagreements or conflicts in recent months because of uncertainty about areas of responsibility?
- If there is no formal structure, do the physicians in your group see a need for a formalized structure?
- Is there agreement on which model should be used?
- Are there any sacred cows (ie, individuals who are often unreasonably immune from criticism or opposition) in the organization? If so, that may cause the best organizational model to be modified.
- Would staff members feel comfortable with the model you are considering?

MISTAKES TO AVOID

- Allowing the organization model to grow by itself
- Failing to design a good model because of personalities

Endnotes

1. Griffith J. *Speakers Library of Stories, Anecdotes and Humor.* Paramus, NJ: Prentice Hall; 1990:363.

2. Mintzberg H. *Mintzberg on Management, Inside Our Strange World of Organizations.* New York, NY: The Free Press; 1989:329.

CHAPTER 4

Writing Useful Job and Process Descriptions

When Drs Mary, Frank, and George combined their individual practices into a group practice, they each had a general idea of how the office would function after the merger. Someone at the front desk would check the patients in and out. Another individual would answer the telephone and book the appointments, and a third person would take care of the billing and insurance. Dr George's bookkeeper, who had been with him for 15 years, could also function as the office manager and take care of daily operations and accounts payable. Each physician was bringing current employees into the new practice, although the partners had not really discussed what role each person would fill. All staff members had already proven themselves to be responsible employees who could get the job done.

In addition to the administrative staff, each physician had a nurse, and all three nurses would come into the new practice. The physicians were using their nurses in varying capacities. Dr Mary had a registered nurse (RN) who placed her patients in an examination room, took their vital signs, and assisted with minor procedures. Dr Mary liked to make return calls to patients herself at the end of the day. Drs Frank and George, on the other hand, expected their nurses to handle the return calls after they had discussed the patient's question.

None of the physicians had found it necessary to have job descriptions in place in solo practice. Everyone in a small office had to learn to do whatever needed to be done. The physicians believed that delineating responsibility would only lead to a "that's not my job" culture—a culture they did not want to foster.

Within a short time, however, it became obvious that things were not working as planned. Dr Frank's nurse believed she was doing more responsible work than Dr Mary's nurse and wanted a salary increase. The receptionist, who was hired for her people skills, was now responsible for posting charges and submitting claims. She had little insurance experience, but she felt that she should be given a raise because of her additional responsibilities. The office manager was overwhelmed by the responsibilities of managing staff in addition to her bookkeeping tasks. Besides, she much preferred working with number problems than with people problems. The physicians agreed they needed help.

LESSONS LEARNED

The practice of Drs Mary, Frank, and George was experiencing the growing pains that many practices go through when circumstances change. Often business decisions overshadow the equally important people decisions. Many solo practitioners believe that since the office is small, formal job descriptions will only get in the way. The informal, unwritten job description is: Do whatever it takes to get the job done. However, lack of structured job outlines can lead to confusion, feelings of being taken advantage of, and important tasks falling through the cracks because no one takes responsibility. To build an outstanding team means starting with each job and achieving the following:

- hiring the best person for the job,
- adding to the individual's knowledge by providing additional job training,
- allowing the individual to grow in the job,
- developing the individual to be able to assume a more responsible job, and
- providing the individual with feedback on how he or she is performing on the job.

To have an outstanding work team, you need to have a clear understanding of what each job entails. Increasingly, however, the need for speed and performance in a job requires flexible job descriptions. Today's employees are expected to engage in multitasking. Some organizations that have adapted total quality management (TQM) and reengineering programs have begun to focus more on the process of the work than on the description of the job.

What are the differences between process-based organizations and more traditional job-based organizations? A key component of a process-based organization is that process descriptions are more fluid, less reliant on printed documentation of a job, and more focused on process descriptions. In a process-based organization, employees are continually questioning the efficiency of the work they perform. In a job-based organization, on the other hand, job descriptions are inclined to be static, with very few changes over time.

In a health care environment, it may be desirable to have the stability of job-based roles with clear lines of responsibility, but to focus on the improvement process as well. Therefore, we are going to combine the two methods of defining roles. The idea is to develop written job descriptions using job analysis and task analysis so that staff members will be able to make improvements as they perform their jobs. The goal is to have the work performed efficiently, to make changes as needed, and to maintain a primary focus on quality patient care.

In the example at the beginning of this chapter, the problems associated with a lack of formalized job descriptions were compounded by the merging of the practices. Problems included workers with the same title (ie, the nurses) having different levels of responsibility, and front office personnel in roles for which they were not best suited—a receptionist performing billing and collections, and a billing and collections person acting as office manager. To make this practice function better will require completing the following steps:

- Assessing the jobs that are currently being performed in the office
- Developing descriptions to describe the responsibilities of the jobs
- Placing the person best suited for each job in the role.

JOB ANALYSIS

Job analysis is the process of gathering, organizing, evaluating, and reporting work-related information. When a job is analyzed, the information can be used to hire the best person, design training for that job, determine compensation, develop the job description, and review the individual's performance.

The first step in successfully developing appropriate job descriptions is to complete a job analysis worksheet. There are three approaches to developing a job analysis worksheet. The first is to interview employees in the job; the second is to observe the employee performing the job; and the third is to briefly perform the job yourself.

In the first approach, the employee provides the needed information by answering a series of questions. **Form 4-1** will assist in analyzing the job. During this process, look for omissions in work flow or related tasks that are not mentioned, and question the staff member about them. This may prompt the staff member to remember forgotten tasks or reveal lapses in job responsibilities.

FORM 4-1. JOB ANALYSIS—EMPLOYEE INTERVIEW

Questions	Responsibilities
What are your primary responsibilities?	1. 2. 3. 4.
What are your secondary responsibilities?	1. 2. 3. 4.
What are your occasional responsibilities?	1. 2. 3. 4.

Task	How often performed?	Length of time needed to perform?	What else is happening when you perform this task?
1. 2. 3. 4. 5. 6. 7.			

In the second approach, the employee is observed while performing the job. Although sitting with the employee for an hour may not reveal all the tasks the employee performs, it will provide firsthand information about the process that is being performed and indicate whether the process is working as efficiently as possible. After completing the observation, the observer should note discrepancies in the reported length of time to complete a task, frequency of tasks, and other contributing factors. Use **Form 4-2** to capture the observation information.

Keep in mind that the employee may perform the job differently when no one is watching. However, an observer can obtain valuable information about a job by witnessing the interactions with other staff members, physicians, and patients. For example, an employee may repeatedly need to take extra time to explain a procedure or policy to a patient. Without firsthand observation, a supervisor may believe that the employee has

FORM 4-2. JOB ANALYSIS—OBSERVATION

What does employee spend the most time doing?	1. 2. 3. 4. 5. 6.
What is the length of time it takes employee to perform each task?	1. 2. 3. 4. 5.
What interruptions/inefficiencies does employee encounter?	Describe:

more free time than actually is the case. This can work conversely as well. The employee may describe tasks in such great detail that a supervisor is led to believe that the employee is overwhelmed with work, when in actuality each task is relatively straightforward and easy to perform.

In the third approach, the supervisor actually performs the job for a short time. This method provides a better picture of the job, the tasks involved, and the primary and secondary responsibilities. The employee, however, must take time to train the observer, and the time commitment is greater than in the first two methods.

Once you have completed two or three approaches, the next step is compiling the information in a job analysis worksheet (**Form 4-3**).

1. In column 1, write down the tasks that the person reports doing on a daily, weekly, monthly, or occasional basis.

2. In column 2, identify other people involved in the process. For example, a patient is involved in almost every function in the office. The appointment scheduler may also have to interact with a physician or nurse in order to perform the task of setting the appointment.

3. In column 3, ask the employee how many times a day that particular task is performed. This will vary depending on the number of patients seen, number of telephone calls taken, or number of lab tests ordered. You should be able to obtain an average number of times the task is performed.

4. Next, in column 4, identify the length of time it takes to perform the task each time it is done. Again, this will vary depending on the

patient or circumstances, but you will have an idea of the length of time it takes to perform the service on the average. This information can be used later to determine whether the expectations of the person performing the job are reasonable, and whether efficiency can be improved.

5. Column 5 leaves room for recording comments as you obtain information. These can be insights the employee provides, or notes from personal observation.

6. Column 6 is a check column. After selecting one of the three methods for performing the job analysis (ie, personal interview, observation, performing the job yourself), it is advisable to cross-check your findings with a second method. For example, a receptionist may tell you that all she does is check patients in when they come into the office, verify their insurance information in the computer, and alert the nurse that the patient is ready. The whole process usually takes 15 to 20 minutes. This may seem like a long time per patient until you observe her also calling insurance companies for preauthorization when a patient fails to bring in this information, answering incoming calls when the telephone receptionist gets backlogged, and tracking down new patient medical records that were forwarded in advance. These additional tasks need to be recorded in the job analysis review. The check column allows you to record additional information discovered from the second method.

FORM 4-3. JOB ANALYSIS—WORKSHEET I

List of tasks employee performs on a weekly/monthly/ occasional basis	What other individuals involved in the process?	How many times a day is the task performed?	How long does it take employee to perform the task on average?	Comments	Additional information
Task 1					
Task 2					
Task 3					
Task 4					
Task 5					

SATISFACTION INDICATORS

The second step in establishing good written job descriptions is to identify potential sources of job satisfaction and job dissatisfaction. For example, a physician's nurse may experience job satisfaction from helping people and providing a service. Job dissatisfaction may result from unpredictable hours and having to work late in the evening. By obtaining these satisfaction indicators, you will have identified areas for improving the job, have a better understanding of what motivates the person in the job, and possibly decide to modify the job to improve the satisfaction level.

The importance of job satisfaction cannot be overstated. People rarely succeed at anything unless they enjoy doing it. Successful managers have discovered that finding good employees and paying them well is not enough to ensure top performance. The person also has to really enjoy the work. It has been said, "Money will buy a good dog, but it won't buy the wag of his tail." To ensure employees are happy in their work, it is important to get an accurate picture of the satisfaction each particular job has to offer. **Form 4-4** captures information about the tools of the job and sources of job satisfaction.

DEVELOPING THE JOB DESCRIPTION

Once the job analysis worksheet has been completed, a job description can be developed (**Form 4-5**). The purpose of a job description is to let employees know the following aspects of their jobs.

- What they are expected to do
- How well they are expected to do it
- How their performance compares to the standards of the job.

Begin the job description process by identifying major performance issues from your analysis worksheet. These performance issues will be used to describe the basic job function and areas of responsibility.

PHYSICAL REQUIREMENTS

The final section of the job description should identify the physical requirements of the job and any exposure to risk. This will assist the practice in adhering to ADA guidelines for hiring and will advise potential applicants of risk involved.

The Americans with Disabilities Act of 1990 (ADA) prohibits employment discrimination against qualified individuals with disabilities and applies to private employers with 15 or more workers. A *disability* under the ADA is defined as a physical or mental impairment that substantially limits one or more major life activities, a history of such impairment, or being regarded as having such an impairment. A *qualified individual* is defined as an individual with a disability who satisfied the requisite skill,

---

FORM 4-4. JOB ANALYSIS—WORKSHEET II

Job Title _____

Grade/Salary Level _____

Position Reports to (Title) _____

Job Information
List the most important duties and responsibilities (typically 5 or 6).

_____
_____
_____
_____

Describe key involvement with superiors, subordinates, peers, vendors, customers, and other contacts.

_____
_____
_____
_____

What are the potential sources of satisfaction? (List up to 5)

_____
_____
_____
_____

What are the potential sources of dissatisfaction? (List up to 5)

_____
_____
_____
_____

What jobs or career opportunities might be available? (Indicate even if limited.)

_____
_____
_____
_____

experience, and educational requirements of an employment position and who *with or without reasonable accommodation* can perform the essential functions of the position.

Reasonable accommodation refers to any change in the work environment or in the customary way of doing things that enables an individual with a disability to perform the functions of a particular job. An employer may not discriminate against a qualified but handicapped

---

FORM 4-5. JOB DESCRIPTION WORKSHEET

Job Title (as it appears on the organization chart or on personnel records)
_____

Basic Job Function (State in one sentence.)
_____
_____
_____
_____

Relationships
Whom does this person report to?   _____
Whom does this person supervise?   _____
Whom does this person work closely with?   _____
What are this person's contacts outside the company? _____

Responsibilities
These will be divided into two groups—primary responsibilities and secondary responsibilities. Condense the tasks you identified on the Job Analysis Worksheet into four or five primary responsibilities and four or five secondary responsibilities.

Primary	Secondary

Performance Standards
The performance standards established in the job description will be used in the performance evaluation. The Job Analysis Worksheet will assist in establishing reasonable performance standards. Below are examples of established standards of performance for a receptionist:

    1. Answer the telephone within three rings.

    2. Identify yourself to caller each time you answer the telephone.

    3. Greet patients within 5 seconds of their walking in the door.

    4. Process all patient registration with a 98% accuracy rate.

Authority: List authority responsibilities and limits. For example:
Can approve purchases up to $500.
Authority to write off accounts up to $100.
Has authority to grant time off.

_____
_____
_____

individual and is required by law to accommodate the physical or mental impairment of a handicapped applicant or employee unless the accommodation would impose an "undue hardship" on the operation of the employer's business. Examples of accommodations include modification of work schedule, physical qualifications, or relocations of particular jobs or offices. Under the ADA, reasonable accommodation can be broken down into three categories:

- the equal opportunity to employment,
- measures that enable a person to perform the job, and
- measures that enable employees with disabilities to enjoy the same benefits and privileges as are enjoyed by other employees.

To comply with these guidelines and ensure that no discrimination takes place in the hiring process, a review of the job to be performed and an inventory of the job's physical requirements can be conducted. Questions regarding the physical requirements of a job may include the following.

- What is the degree of physical exertion (light, moderate, heavy)?
- What body positions or movements are required to do the job (sitting, standing, walking, reaching, stooping, sensing/feeling)?
- What object manipulation is required (grasping the telephone/placing a needle in a vein)?
- What is required visually (a keen sense of vision or little visual ability)?

Once job requirements have been identified and included in the job description, interviewers can hand all applicants a copy of the job description. After asking each applicant to review the job requirements, the interviewer can then ask the individual if he or she can perform the job as stated. If the applicant indicates that he or she could not due to a disability or handicap, the interviewer can ask what modifications could be made for him or her to perform the job. Again as a reminder, the employer is expected to make reasonable accommodations that would not cause undue hardship on the business. For example, a nurse may need to be able to lift up to 50 pounds, stand for long periods of time, and be able to converse with patients. There is some risk of exposure to disease. Job description software programs are available that can lead you through this part of the development process.

JOB CONTENT REVIEW

The final step is to review the job process descriptions periodically to reestablish their legitimacy and to ensure control over job content. Job content should do the following.

- Safeguard funds. For example, a single person should not handle all the financial functions; instead separation of responsibilities should be established.
- Reflect change in workload and job tasks as the practice grows and changes. Many times, job descriptions are designed when a practice is established or a new job is created and not looked at again. Job and process descriptions should be living documents, with modified descriptions to reflect each job as it is today.
- Increase employee satisfaction. As you complete your job analysis worksheet, it is important to pay special attention to the potential sources of satisfaction. If you cannot identify good sources for job satisfaction or have difficulty doing so, it is time to consider revising the job description. To increase employee retention and longevity, job satisfaction is high on the list.

In addition to acting as a tool in hiring new employees and providing performance standards to be used in evaluations, job descriptions can be used to review staff structure and the distribution of work. Frequently, as a medical practice evolves, responsibilities may be assigned to certain individuals because of a lack of alternatives. Rather than assigning tasks to the person best suited for performing them, they often are assigned to the person with the most available time. In analyzing the operations of the practice, consider the following questions.

- Are there any inconsistencies in job titles and responsibility? An example would be a receptionist who posts EOBs or an office manager who provides backup telephone coverage. In such cases, consider reassigning the task to the person with the appropriate job title. If the person performing the task is capable, but the job title does not reflect the level of responsibility, consider changing job titles and raising the pay of the person according to the job responsibilities.
- Do jobs requiring people skills belong to the staff members who have people skills? The office manager's dilemma is when a good technical person is in a people skills job. If the employee exhibits both good technical and interpersonal skills, make every effort to retain the individual. If, on the other hand, the employee does not have the skills

to deal with patients with the finesse you expect, reassign the employee at once.

- What is consuming each employee's time? Is it the major job requirements or dozens of menial tasks? If you find that minor tasks are eating up the employee's workday, ask whether the minor tasks need to be done on a daily basis; if someone else is better suited to do them; if part of the task can be eliminated to reduce the amount of time spent; and if additional staff is required.
- What tasks are not being done that need to be done? It happens in every office—some important tasks just never seem to get accomplished. Those tasks vary from sorting magazines in the examination rooms, to calling patients about their accounts, to filing incoming lab results in the patients' records. By identifying tasks that are often put off or ignored, giving them an importance rating (eg, on a scale of 1 to 5, with 1 being of very little importance and 5 being highly important), you can determine where to refocus assignments. Tasks with a rating of 5 must be placed at the top of someone's list.

Evaluation of tasks and processes should be performed before any major changes in staffing (such as creating a new position or reengineering the organization) take place. The analysis can also be performed when someone leaves the organization and as you begin the search for a replacement. The management time invested in this phase of the employee selection process will facilitate finding the best person for the job. Once developed, the job description will be useful in recruiting, developing effective performance evaluations, evaluating pay rates, hiring the best person, and developing a training program.

MISTAKES TO AVOID

- Not reviewing job descriptions periodically
- Believing that employees know job responsibilities and performance standards
- Believing that job descriptions are not needed

Endnote

1. Aspen Health Law Center Aspen Reference Group. *Medical Group Practice Legal and Administrative Guide.* Gaithersburg, Md: Aspen Publications; 1998:33-34.

CHAPTER 5

Recruiting the People You Want on Your Team

W hen Susan accepted the position of office manager for a four-physician practice, she discovered that she also inherited the responsibility of filling three job openings. The practice had experienced turnover when the former office manager left, and it was Susan's job to fill openings for a nurse, a receptionist, and a billing specialist as quickly as possible. Feeling slightly overwhelmed by the tasks at hand, Susan decided to hire people as quickly as possible. She placed advertisements in the classified section of the local newspaper. The ads read as follows:

Wanted: [Nurse] for physicians' practice. Very busy practice needs [nurse to assist physician with patient care]. Convenient location. Excellent benefits. Please call (555) 555-5555.

Susan received many calls about the openings and spent considerable time screening applicants to eliminate those who did not have the skills to perform the job. She finally hired a billing specialist who was a friend of another billing specialist, taking the staff member's word that the person could do the job. She filled the nurse and receptionist positions with people who responded to the advertisements. Then she crossed her fingers, hoped for the best, and went on to other pressing job responsibilities.

Within the first month, however, Susan discovered that the receptionist was overwhelmed by the responsibilities of her position. Although she had experience as a front desk receptionist, she had worked in a smaller office with fewer people to process each day. She was not used to the hectic pace of a four-physician group or the more businesslike culture of the practice. The nurse seemed to be working out well. However, the billing specialist did not have the experience Susan hoped she had. The friend who had recommended her was having to do more work to make up for the deficit. Within 2 months, Susan faced the task of hiring another billing specialist and receptionist.

LESSONS LEARNED

Although Susan was an experienced and successful office manager, she succumbed to the "let's-fill-the-openings-as-quickly-as-possible" method of hiring new staff members. She made three management errors that resulted in her having to do the job again.

Her first error was in not assessing the job responsibilities of the openings she was trying to fill. She let job titles rather than job descriptions drive her recruiting methods and her decisions. Therefore, she ended up with people who could not perform all the duties the jobs required. While hiring less experienced people and training them is always an option, Susan had not considered offering training to the new staff members. She focused on people she believed would require no training. After all, she was overwhelmed. She did not need the added responsibilities of training. Neither had she considered the unique culture of the organization and assessed how candidates would fit in their new environment.

Second, Susan did not tailor her newspaper advertising to specifically target people with the skills, behaviors, and experience that she wanted. Her generic ads resulted in her having to spend more time screening the initial calls before focusing on viable candidates.

Third, while word-of-mouth recruiting is often a good way to find new employees, Susan should have interviewed the billing specialist who was recommended by an employee, using the same interviewing steps that she would have used with any other applicant.

Like Susan, office managers, administrators, and physicians often find themselves desperately seeking good people to fill vacant positions while they are overloaded with work themselves. In their haste to fill the vacancies, they often make recruiting and hiring mistakes. To avoid those mistakes and find the right people for the right job, two rules must be followed.

First, develop a clear picture of exactly the type of person for whom you are looking.

- What will this person have to do?
- How much experience will he or she need?
- Are you willing to train?
- How much training are you willing to provide?

- Does the person need to be able to interact with patients, or will the person always be away from the action?
- Does the person need to be detail oriented and focused on the task at hand, or able to handle many tasks at once?
- Does the person need to display initiative and take the lead, or take direction easily?
- Does the person need to work with someone who is a perfectionist or micromanager, or will the person manage himself or herself?

Second, to develop a precise idea of what you are looking for, assess the following three job components:

- the knowledge, skill, and abilities that are required to do the job,
- the behavior you want to see from the person who holds that job, and
- the environmental issues associated with the job.

You can obtain this information from paper sources and from people sources. The paper sources are the job analysis worksheet, the satisfaction indicator analysis, the job description you developed, and performance evaluations of employees who have held that job in the past. The people sources are employees who have worked in the position, supervisors, peers, incumbents, and, of course, yourself.

GATHERING INFORMATION FROM PAPER SOURCES

To develop a picture of your ideal candidate using paper sources, gather the sources and go through them carefully. Highlight areas that describe the employee's knowledge, technical skills, education, and experience. These factors will help determine whether a candidate will be able to do the job. For each candidate, develop a grid that lists identified factors, such as the one in **Form 5-1.**

FORM 5-1. CANDIDATE ABILITIES GRID

Knowledge	Skills	Abilities

Next, use a second color to highlight the behaviors you expect from a person holding that job. You may have labeled the behaviors with terms such as *industrious, dependable, detail oriented, courteous,* and *motivated.*

Once you have identified the behaviors, translate them into what you actually mean when you use the words. For example, if you want someone who is *industrious,* ask yourself what you really mean by *industrious.* How would you identify an industrious person? The answer may be that you expect someone who will do the tasks listed in the job description but will also routinely go beyond that job description. Identify someone in your organization who demonstrated that behavior in the past: "I want someone like the kindergarten teacher who we hired part-time in medical records to file incoming labs. She also developed an ideal sample chart and posted it in the medical records department for other new hires and temporary help. That is what industrious means to me." Use a grid similar to the one in **Form 5-2** to help gather the information.

FORM 5-2. BEHAVIOR GRID

1.	Example:
2.	Example:
3.	Example:
4.	Example:
5.	Example:

GATHERING INFORMATION FROM PEOPLE SOURCES

While the people sources can supplement and augment the information gathered from the paper sources, the real value of people sources is to provide information on the environmental issues of the job. Identifying these issues will help determine whether a person will be able to adapt to your workplace.

Environmental issues can range from overall culture to what kind of work space the employee will have. For example, a person who has worked in a large corporate environment with many layers of management where one could almost get lost in the corporation may find the structure of a medical practice too focused or intense. Some environmental issues you might want to consider are as follows.

- What is the decision-making process for this job? Is the person relatively free to decide to make changes, or does it require six people to sign off on a simple decision?
- What kind of work space is available—private office, cubicle, workstation, lab counter shared with others?
- Will this job require the person to take calls or carry a pager?
- Is evening and/or weekend work required?
- Are the hours always the same, or do they vary?
- Does the office close for lunch with telephones forwarded to an answering service, or does the office remain open with staggered lunch hours?
- Do lunch hours sometimes turn into lunch minutes?
- What are the temperaments of the physicians in the group?
- Is the office fast-paced, or are there slow days when the physician is in surgery or out of the office?
- How often is there time to catch up?
- Do the physicians value continuing education for staff members?
- What problems have there been in the past with employees and the environment?

Once these environmental issues are identified, you can translate your findings into a job requirement worksheet (**Form 5-3**).

FORM 5-3. JOB REQUIREMENT WORKSHEET

Knowledge, Skills, and Abilities	Behaviors	Environmental Issues

RECRUITING CANDIDATES

When the worksheet has been completed, the next step is to attract applicants who are likely to have the required skills and desired behaviors, who will find the environment attractive, and who will want to work for you. The idea is to conduct your recruiting campaign to attract only that type of person.

Several recruiting methods are available for finding the most desirable candidates, including word of mouth, newspapers, trade journals and newsletters, and placement agencies. Each method has advantages and disadvantages, and often the best recruiting strategy is to use a combination of methods.

Word-of-mouth recruiting is always a good way to find qualified people. The employees who are already working for you will not want to work with someone who is lazy or incompetent, so they will probably not recommend someone they know is not a good worker. Another advantage is that word-of-mouth recruiting may attract good people who would not otherwise be looking to move. When they hear of your job opening from a friend or contact, they may be prompted to consider making a change. One disadvantage of word-of-mouth recruiting is that an applicant may feel indebted to and feel more allegiance to the friend than they do to the employer.

Newspaper advertising is the most commonly used form of recruiting. It has the advantage of reaching many people who are looking for jobs. The disadvantage is that an ad can generate a low proportion of useful resumes.

Trade journals and newsletters are another means of attracting viable candidates. The advantage of this method is that it targets people already in the field with the skill sets you are seeking. Like word-of-mouth recruiting, an ad in a trade publication may attract people who are not really looking for a change. The disadvantage of using trade journals and newsletters is that it takes more lead time to place an advertisement, and responses may trickle in for a month or more. The ad may also attract people from out of state who will need to relocate.

Placement agencies are often used to find viable candidates. A good agency will conduct a comprehensive recruiting campaign to find a person who fits the requirements. The advantage to using an agency is that most of the screening work is done by someone else, thus relieving the manager of the task of weeding out people who will are not a good fit. Better agencies can determine exactly what an organization is looking for and present two or three qualified people for you to interview. Most agencies allow the employer a 30- to 90-day window to try the person before making a full commitment. The disadvantage of using an agency is that the fees associated with placement are usually a percentage of the individual's salary, which can result in a few thousand dollars. However, much of the time-consuming screening is done by the agency, references are checked, and no payment is due until placement is made.

WRITING THE AD

Whether you choose to fill a job vacancy by word of mouth, direct advertising, or the use of an agency, it's a good idea to develop the ad first and use it for the entire recruiting process.

Imagine for a moment that you are an excellent candidate for a job in a medical practice. Would the ad in **Figure 5-1** catch your eye? Probably not, especially if there were other ads from which to choose, such as the one in **Figure 5-2.** Writing an ad that grabs the reader's attention, delivers your message clearly, and specifies the qualifications you are seeking will help bring the desired results.

There are 10 steps to writing an ad that will attract the kind of job applicants you are looking for.

1. Define the job in as specific terms as possible. You have specific terms defined on your worksheet. If you are looking for a receptionist, write specific responsibilities of that job:

    Receptionist wanted for patient check-in. Job responsibilities include obtaining patient demographics, preparing patient chart, and entering information into the billing system. Position entails verifying insurance, calling for precertifications and authorizations, and setting appointments.

2. Include the technical requirements of the job. Make sure that the listed requirements are in fact needed to perform the job:

    Applicant must have working knowledge of ABC computer system, be familiar with managed care plans in the area, and have working knowledge of HMO and PPO requirements.

FIGURE 5-1. SAMPLE ADVERTISEMENT I

> **MEDICAL OFFICE**
> Full-time, experienced nurse.
> Send resume to G-11 Journal.

FIGURE 5-2. SAMPLE ADVERTISEMENT II

> **DO YOU LOVE KIDS?**
> Our growing, four-doctor pediatric practice is looking for a hardworking, pediatric nurse to help manage a steady flow of patients. We are a fast-paced, busy practice, located in a bright, modern office on the north side. Salary up to _____ , depending on experience. Call _____ at _____ for more information, or forward your resume to _____.

3. State hours, days of week, location, travel, and overtime. Specify all of the environmental factors that will be of importance to an applicant:

   Convenient location near XYZ Corporation. Hours are M-F from 8 am to 5 pm. Occasional overtime is expected.

4. State salary range. Arguments can be made both for and against printing the salary of the job. Providing the salary will prevent calls from people who are looking for considerably more than the job pays.

5. Describe the benefits. Most practices offer about the same benefits. You may want to list them, or merely write something like "Usual Benefits," "Excellent Benefits," or "Competitive Benefit Package."

6. State that you are an Equal Opportunity Employer. A simple EOE will inform applicants that you are an equal opportunity employer.

7. Give information on where to apply:

   Fax resumes to Attn: Human Resources Department at 555-217-2122 or e-mail to HR@Mdoffice.com.

8. Write the ad incorporating all the listed information. It is better to write the ad first to see how much space you will need to buy rather than trying to fit the ad into the space that costs what you want to spend. As one office manager says, "Cutting down on advertising to save money is like stopping your watch to save time." Invest in a well-worded ad and the interview time will be cut in half.

9. Be innovative. Remember, you are contending with every other medical practice and facility in your area for top candidates. In addition, many people working in the medical field leave health care to take jobs in other fields or industries. Your ad must stand out to attract the good candidates.

10. Read your ad as if you were a candidate seeking employment. What does your ad say about you? Does it look stiff and formal, indicating a rigid work environment? Have you sacrificed professionalism in an attempt to be innovative? Does the ad reach out and cause you to want to respond immediately because you are sure this wonderful job was meant for you?

In summary, successful recruiting begins by identifying the skills and behavior that you are looking for in a candidate. You then need to clearly articulate those requirements in well-written ads provided to friends and acquaintances of prospective candidates, and to the agency with which you are working, so that the ideal candidate will be attracted to the job and respond at once.

MISTAKES TO AVOID

- Hiring quickly without doing the homework
- Hiring people to fit the job title rather than the job functions
- Failing to put equal emphasis on job skills, behavioral traits, and environmental issues when hiring

CHAPTER 6

Hiring the Best

When Jill, the office manager of Prime Care, had to recruit a new medical assistant for an opening in the main office, she specified in the ad that the applicant must have a current medical assistant certificate and a minimum of 2 years of experience working in a medical practice. Jill received numerous resumes and eliminated those that did not indicate 2 years of experience. However, her efforts to find the right person for the job kept leading to a dead end.

In desperation, Jill went back through the resumes looking for a qualified assistant with less than 2 years of experience. That is when she came across Stacy's resume. Stacy had good work experience, but had only recently received her medical assistant certificate. Jill was reluctant to call her in for an interview, but did so out of desperation.

During the interview, Stacy's answers revealed a strong work ethic, a commitment to quality, and a willingness to do whatever was needed to get the job done. Jill still preferred to find someone who had worked in a medical practice and would require less training, so she continued her search.

Stacy had decided that Prime Care was the place she wanted to work. She knew she could do the job if given a chance, and she felt she would be comfortable in the work environment. She called Jill after several days to express her interest in the job and asked to be considered despite her lack of experience. She furnished references from her current position as cashier in a grocery store, where she had proven herself to be a conscientious worker. She also furnished the names of references who could attest to her customer service talents—real customers from the grocery store who verified that Stacy had always gone out of her way to be cheerful and helpful. Jill reconsidered, based on the glowing references, and offered Stacy the job. She would later tell anyone who would listen that this was one of the best hiring decisions she ever made.

LESSONS LEARNED

While Stacy required more technical training than an experienced medical assistant, her people skills, work ethic, and attitude helped her become a productive employee almost immediately. Jill decided that from then on, she would not base her hiring decisions primarily on technical skills, but rather on a combination of knowledge, behavior, and the fit of the candidate with the position.

Jill learned an important lesson—do not hire by skills alone. Of all the components involved in the makeup of a good employee (ie, technical skills, behaviors, values, and cultural fit), the technical skills are the easiest to assess and the easiest to change. The more intangible assets of a candidate, on the other hand, are not easily modified and are often difficult to assess. Therefore, effective interviewing skills, assessment tools, reference-checking, and on-the-job assessment should be conducted to verify that an individual is the right one to become part of your organizational family.

Use the job requirement worksheet developed in Chapter 5 to outline the tasks and behaviors that are desired or must be present in the person you hire. Answer the following three questions before hiring a candidate:

1. Can the candidate do the job?
2. Will the candidate do the job?
3. Will the candidate fit into your organization?

QUALIFYING THE CANDIDATE

Like Jill, many people make hiring decisions based primarily on a candidate's education and skills and sometimes overlook the other important components of successful hiring—the behavior of the individual and whether the person will fit into the organization. Of course, no one wants blood drawn by a person who has never performed a venipuncture or an x-ray taken by a technician with no experience. Some technical or educational requirements are mandatory for almost every position in a medical office. However, you can usually be flexible about some points. You can determine which of the candidates you are going to consider by following a series of qualifier steps.

- Step 1: Review the resumes.
- Step 2: Conduct a telephone interview.
- Step 3: Conduct a personal interview (or interviews).
- Step 4: Evaluate the candidate, using assessment tools.
- Step 5: Check references.
- Step 6: Offer trial workdays.

The first step in the employee selection process is to review the resumes that have been submitted. Not every person who submits a resume will progress to a personal interview. If you use a recruiting or employment firm, this part of the employee selection process will be done for you. If you choose to do your own recruiting, you will need to review each resume submitted to determine which candidates possess the required knowledge and skills.

If the position requires a degree, certificate, license, or specific length of time in a former position, you can usually gather such information from the resume. You can also tell if the candidate appears inclined to move from one job to another frequently, to take jobs in different fields for short periods, or to stay with a job. However, it has been said that no one comes so close to perfection as on their resume or job application. Therefore, the assumption is that the only absolutely accurate resume is one that contains no information.

Resume Review

Those applicants whose resumes have passed the initial screening will progress to the telephone screening stage. This process can be a valuable tool not only for screening out unqualified applicants, but also for providing additional insight into the skills and behaviors of viable candidates. By having a set of prepared questions, you ensure that you are fair in the interview process, and that you have not projected the answers you want to hear on one candidate in preference to another. You also ensure that you use the same criteria to evaluate each candidate.

The telephone interview can be used to verify the presence or absence of skills, experience, and education. It can also be an opportunity to address the behaviors you are seeking. In the telephone-screening interview, a set series of four to six questions is asked of each candidate. Only those who have answered all of the questions in the affirmative and have cited a concrete example should be considered for a personal interview. The purpose of this interview is to help you focus on the presence or absence of behaviors. It requires careful listening and staying tuned to what the applicant is saying.

Telephone Interview

For example, say you are looking for a new supervisor for your clinical staff, and you have identified the job knowledge factors as follows.

- Current nursing license
- Minimum of 5 years working experience in a medical office
- Minimum of 2 years of experience supervising others

The environmental issues are as follows.

- Will be required to oversee one person in a satellite location
- Position involves staffing the office for Saturday morning clinic
- Will occasionally need to stay late
- Will work in an office that is quite small

Behavioral characteristics for this supervisor are as follows.

- Must be enthusiastic about the work
- Should be able to inspire enthusiasm in others
- Makes employees feel comfortable about approaching with questions
- Displays tact and diplomacy in dealing with others
- Relates well to physicians, employees, and patients

The list of telephone interview questions for a person in this supervisory position might look like those in **Table 6-1.**

TABLE 6-1. TELEPHONE INTERVIEW QUESTIONS

Questions	Desired Answers
1. Do you like to work? Why did you leave (or are you leaving) your previous position?	Yes
2. Do other people regularly come to you for advice? (If yes, please give an example.)	Yes
3. Do you do something at work better than anyone else? (If yes, what is it that you do better than anyone else?)	Yes
4. Have you given positive recognition to another person within the past 2 weeks? (If yes, give an example.)	Yes
5. Have you developed enthusiasm in other people within the past 2 weeks? (If yes, how did you develop this enthusiasm?)	Yes
6. Are you considerate of others' feelings? (If yes, please give an example.)	Yes

The key to successful telephone interviews is to identify the behavioral characteristics you seek, and then to listen carefully to exact examples of how a candidate has displayed such characteristics. Generalized statements such as "I enjoy working with people" are meaningless unless the applicant can demonstrate how he or she enjoys working with people. The applicant might say, "I love working in a team environment where you work really hard during the day, but share a sense of accomplishment at the end of the day." Another example would be, "I really enjoy helping the elderly patients as they come into the office. Many of them do not have anyone else to listen to them, and I feel that is something I can do." By the time you have completed the telephone interview process, you should be able to narrow the file to two or three good candidates for the personal interview.

Personal Interview

A personal interview is very much like a first date. Both parties put on their best faces and hope to make a good impression. Just like other first dates, the more comfortable a person is, the more the person will be willing to reveal. That is the key to conducting an effective interview. It is important to have the candidate relax, open up, and begin to reveal his or her real character. Therefore, your job is to conduct the interview in a conversational tone in a relatively informal space that will nurture a sense of mutual trust and respect.

Creating this relaxed atmosphere takes time. It is difficult to reach the stage of openness if you have only 30 minutes for the interview and you are interrupted two times. Set aside enough time for an effective interview and ask that there not be interruptions.

Next, create a comfortable atmosphere. You may not have a private office with a cozy corner (few medical office managers do), so find a space that comes as close as possible. That may mean borrowing a physician's office, hiding the stacks of paper under the desk to make the office presentable, or meeting the applicant after hours.

The seating arrangement during the interview is as important as the room itself. Interviewing across a desk is like interviewing across a moat. It decreases communication and prevents the conversational tone that promotes comfort and rapport. Chairs placed at right angles will better facilitate conversation and make it appear that the candidate is a guest rather than the object of an interrogation. Taking time to build the right atmosphere can help you gather better data, promote more open responses from the candidate, project a positive image of the organization, and increase the candidates' accept rate (ie, the percentage of people who accept a position with the organization once you have made a job offer).

Develop a standard set of questions for the personal interview. The questions should help you determine if the candidate can do the job, will do the job, and will fit into your organization. The questions will focus your attention on more important issues and ensure that you have given each applicant the same consideration. Questions should be easy to ask and answer. They should appear to be casual. They should not telegraph what qualities you are looking for. And they should be easy to follow up on to get more detail.

The goal of the personal interview is to build positive rapport, which will give you the opportunity to get details not ordinarily available. What happens during the first 30 to 60 seconds of the interview is vital to setting the stage for the entire meeting. You want to create an atmosphere of spontaneity and help the applicant overcome initial awkwardness. Therefore, when you first meet the applicant, call him or her by name (Ms White). Introduce yourself ("I'm Jane Brown, the office manager"), and thank the applicant for coming. Make small talk to relax the applicant ("Did you have any trouble finding us?" "It looks like we're having an early spring, doesn't it?").

Once the initial small talk has established a relaxed feeling, a natural transition to the prepared questions will lead the candidate to respond in an open manner. Go over the candidate's work experience, educational background, outside interests and activities, and conclude with the self-assessment.

Avoid questions of a personal nature that potentially violate a candidate's rights (eg, do you have children, are you married, do you own a car). To find out if the applicant can meet the job requirements, state the requirement as clearly as possible and then ask a close-ended question. "This job often entails working until 6 or 7 o'clock in the evening, so let me ask you if you are aware of anything that would prevent you from meeting this requirement." The same question should be asked of all candidates, and the candidate should be advised that negative answers are being documented. If other members of the staff participate in the interview process, make sure they are also aware of legal issues in the interview process.

Once you have obtained information about the candidate, present information about the organization—the job, benefits, training, salary, and how quickly you hope to fill the position. Ask the candidate if there are questions, and then review the next steps in the interview process. When this is completed, the interview is over. Thank the candidate for coming, and walk him or her out. Then complete a summary statement about the candidate and determine whether you are interested in making the candidate a job offer.

In some cases, the candidate may meet a panel of interviewers, meet with key people consecutively, or return for a second round of interviews. It is advisable to obtain at least one other person's input for the hiring process. You may prefer to interview all candidates on the first round, and then ask them back for a second interview with someone else in the organization. The second date always reveals more about the person than you saw during the first. If during the second interview your conclusions from the first session are confirmed, then you can trust your initial summary.

EVALUATING THE CANDIDATE WITH ASSESSMENT TOOLS

When you have completed the interview process, the next step is to assess the skills and behaviors of the candidates. Pre-employment testing helps differentiate between candidates possessing the knowledge, skills, and behaviors that will benefit the practice, and those who merely claim to have these qualities. Experts say that testing can reduce turnover by as much as 25%. By assessing skills and behaviors, you can eliminate unsuitable candidates without wasting valuable time in a trial employment period.

When using assessment tools, there are three basic options: (1) designing your own tests, (2) purchasing existing tests, and (3) contracting with an agency to perform the screening. If the practice chooses to design its own assessment tool, it should keep the questions job-related. Devise tests to simulate the actual job the applicant will be doing. Administering assessment tests is legal as long as the tests are conducted fairly and actually pertain to the open position. Therefore, it is reasonable to test a medical records file clerk on speed and accuracy of putting a list in alphabetical order, but it would not be reasonable to expect this candidate to know coding and billing (unless these were part of the job). Likewise, it would be advantageous to test a billing supervisor's skills in Medicare and Medicaid regulations and coding and billing, but it would not be appropriate to include medical questions. It may be advisable to have your assessment tools reviewed by legal counsel before implementing them.

Employees presently holding the job will be able to help design an assessment tool for their position. Once the test is designed, implement it and track the results to determine whether employees who perform well on the test actually perform well on the job, turnover decreases, and new hires require less training time than before.

If you prefer to use standardized tests from existing packages, find a test pertinent to the job and administer tests consistently to each candidate.

When using assessment tools, bear in mind that you want to assess not only the candidate's skills, but also their behaviors. Relationships, skills, attitude, and motivation should be assessed prior to hiring. There are assessment tools on the market for evaluating behaviors, as well as firms that specialize in administering tests and conducting interviews to assess the behaviors and values of a candidate.

While most managers know the importance of hiring the person with the right skills, many are inclined to make the mistake of relying on intuition to make a hiring decision. The trouble with this method is that you may like the candidate personally, and you may thus hire someone who isn't suited for the job. People tend to like other people who are similar to themselves. If you hire based on this, you will end up with an entire staff like you—with the same strengths and weaknesses. What you really want to determine is whether the candidate can help move your organization to a higher level of performance; whether you can rely on the new hire to be self-motivated; whether the employee will be able to move from a staff position to a leadership role; and whether the employee can adapt to the changing health care environment.

REFERENCE CHECKS

The final step before making an offer to a candidate is to check references. Many times, reference checks reveal important information that did not come out in the interview.

Since many former employers are aware of the legal repercussions of giving a bad reference, they may be reluctant to provide information. Although many organizations will only confirm dates of service, it is usually possible to find someone (such as a former supervisor or physician) who will be willing to give a reference. Obtaining a signed agreement from the prospective employee giving the former employer authorization to release information, and submitting your request in writing, may produce results.

It is often necessary in reference checks to read between the lines and hear what is not said as well as what is. One physician was hesitant to hire an applicant because the answer to the question, "Was she a good employee?" brought the response, "Yes, she was pretty good." The physician had hoped to hear what he had heard in the past about outstanding employees, which was something to the effect of, "Yes, indeed. She's the best I ever had." When he did not hear those words, he doubted if the candidate was really the one he wanted to hire. He did hire her, to discover that the reference was accurate in that she was only "a pretty good employee." One former employer responded to the question, "Is he steady?" by saying, "Heck yes, he's steady. He's practically motionless."

Besides providing better insight about a candidate, well-documented reference checks will protect you in the event you make a hiring mistake. Under the doctrine of *respondeat superior,* the employer is responsible for the harm committed by its employees acting within the scope of their employment. This harm can range from billing and coding incorrectly to giving out erroneous information or being negligent.

In addition to the doctrine of *respondeat superior,* some states recognize a cause for action for negligent hiring. Under such a cause of action, an employer may be liable for the tortuous or even criminal acts of its employees when the employer breaches its duty of care in hiring competent employees. That is, when an employer knew or should have known through the exercise of reasonable diligence that an employee poses an unreasonable risk of harm to others.

Negligent hiring claims may be filed by coemployees, clients, patients, or even members of the public at large. These claims typically involve personal injuries arising out of an assault and battery, accident, theft, or sexual harassment. Plaintiffs may be awarded compensatory and punitive damages. Due to the possibility of suits resulting from hiring "the wrong person," reference checks have become critical to the hiring process. The information received through the reference check should be documented and include the date of the reference check, the name of the individual soliciting the information on behalf of the prospective employer, the name of the person providing the information from the past employer, and a detailed description of the information communicated. Even if the past employer refuses to provide information or provides only "name, rank and serial number," that information should be recorded.[1]

The Office of Inspector General's model compliance plans provide another reason for performing reference and background checks on prospective employees. Health care organizations are encouraged to perform background checks on those people hired who may be in a position of discretionary authority.

TRIAL DAYS

Some practices offer candidates an opportunity to work trial days, or to do or observe the job for a short period before accepting the job offer. This allows the candidate to evaluate the culture of the firm, the working conditions, and the work itself. Trial days help a candidate determine if the job is suitable; this in turn helps minimize turnover.

MISTAKES TO AVOID

- Doing most of the talking during the interview
- Letting personal likes and dislikes interfere with an assessment
- Hiring by intuition

Endnote
1. Flax JP. *Employment Issues in the Workplace.* Atlanta, Ga: Alston & Bird LLP; March 2000.

CHAPTER 7

Training and Development

When Melinda joined the Midtown Cardiology Associates central billing office, she brought more than 7 years experience in billing and collections to her new position. In fact, her prior work experience was so good that her new manager thought it would be an insult to show her how to do things. So, after she showed Melinda where the coffeepot, copier, and restrooms were and gave her a hurried overview of the job, the manager pretty much left Melinda alone.

Melinda felt a little overwhelmed the first day as she tried to determine who reported to whom, which managed care plans the physicians were participating in, and how work flowed through the practice. As the weeks passed, her feelings of being overwhelmed turned into feelings of frustration. She could sense impatience on the part of her coworkers when she made mistakes, and they occasionally admonished her, saying "You should know that by now," and "We don't do things like that here." Melinda felt like she had failed; her supervisor was unhappy with her progress; and eventually Melinda left for another job. Her on-the-job training had turned out to be the bits and pieces of information she was able to pick up from helpful coworkers.

LESSONS LEARNED

One of the most important responsibilities of any manager is training and developing the staff. Only with well-trained staff members will a practice achieve its objectives. Unfortunately, this is one of the areas where managers often focus the least attention, relying instead on an employee's past experience and education as a substitute for training.

But whether employees are new to the work force, new to the profession, or have 20 years experience in the field, they will always need ongoing training and development to help them be the best they can be. Medicine is changing, the health care environment is changing, people are changing, and the business world is changing. Ongoing education and development to keep abreast of these changes is an absolute necessity for a practice to thrive.

Unfortunately, few practices have the luxury of employing a full-time trainer. Therefore, the responsibility of training and development often falls on the manager or on other employees designated by the manager.

THE TRAINING PROCESS

Training is usually required at three critical points in an employee's tenure with an organization: (1) when the employee is first hired, (2) when there are new developments in the field, and (3) when the employee assumes new responsibilities. Employees usually receive some training at these critical times. Rarely is an employee thrown into the job without some type of orientation, even if that consists of saying, "Here, sit next to Linda, and she'll tell you what to do." Sometimes the training is every bit that extensive when an individual is asked to assume additional responsibilities or is moved to a new job.

Training must also be timely. Sending someone to a class about something they're not going to have to do until next year is not the best use of training dollars. When the time comes to use the new skills, the employee either will have forgotten them or will have lost enthusiasm for the work. Training needs to be conducted so that the employee is able to carry the new skills over into the job.

Once an employee has received training, it is important to allow the employee to begin using it immediately to increase retention. An exercise that will increase employee retention is to have the person give a mini-training session to coworkers. Other department members will then also benefit from the training investment. Building an effective training program will help with employee morale and retention, produce a better product, and contribute to the practice's success.

To determine where and how many training dollars will be invested, complete the following exercise. Set aside an annual training budget. This can be a percentage of staff salaries to be figured into personnel costs, a percentage of revenue, or a set dollar amount. Then determine what the overall training needs of the organization are. Often the individuals who are bold enough to request training are the ones to receive it. By determining first where training is needed, you will be able to direct your dollars where they will do the most good. Ask whether staff members need training in improving supervisory skills, coding and government regulations, accounts receivable management, the patient encounter and improving patient satisfaction, or ongoing training for licensure or recertification.

Once you have made these decisions, the next step is to determine where the best training for the dollar can be found. Is the hospital planning on offering training in these areas? Are there practice management associates or coding associates who will be addressing these topics? Is there Web-based training available on these topics? Will Web-based training satisfy staff members' needs, or would interactive participation be better?

As a manager, you can build a winning team by taking four quality improvement steps. Step 1 is to select the individual based on talent and abilities. Step 2 is to provide comprehensive orientation. Step 3 is to follow a training certification process. Step 4 is to develop an ongoing learning environment.

ORIENTATION

Step 1 was addressed in Chapter 6. By following the advice in that chapter, you have hired the best applicant based on talent and abilities. Developing your employee-training program will fulfill steps 2, 3, and 4. Begin with employee orientation.

Do you remember your first day on the job? How did you feel when you walked in the door? There are so many things that contribute to the anxiety of beginning a new job. Where are the restrooms? When and where do I have lunch? Whom am I sitting next to? What is my supervisor like? Will my supervisor and coworkers like me? Will I fit in? Did I make the right choice?

A new employee will not be able to start focusing on the job until those questions are answered. Therefore, be proactive and address the issues immediately. A formal training program will ensure that you or the person you assigned to conduct the orientation will cover all the subjects and allow the employee time to ask additional questions.

Form 7-1 is a sample orientation plan. Each item is checked off as it is addressed. When the orientation list has been completed, the trainer can sign off on the checklist, which becomes part of the employee's record. It serves as a written record that the new employee was informed, for example, that no one is to enter the office after hours without prior permission.

However, going over all issues at once and documenting that issues were addressed does not mean that a new employee has comprehended and retained all the information. Therefore, a series of follow-up test questions should be developed to ensure that the individual fully

FORM 7-1. SAMPLE ORIENTATION

Topic	Orientation completed by	Date
Information About the Practice		
History of the organization		
Biographical sketch of physicians and their areas of expertise		
Mission and value of the practice		
Number of employees and locations of other offices		
Organizational chart and reporting lines that describe the practice structure		
What level of service do you expect for your patients		
Information About the Working Environment		
Tour of facility		
Types of correspondence and approval for each (memo, e-mail, etc)		
Dress code		
Identification badge, building pass, parking pass		
Policy for entering the building after hours		
Security and safety issues		
Refrigerator policies		
Selling of fund-raising or other goods		
Information Handbook		
Personnel policies		
OSHA training		
Hazardous communication training		
Compliance training		
Release of confidential information		

understands your policies on entering the building after hours, sending out e-mail or memos without approval, and releasing patient information. The tests can be broken into segments. See **Tables 7-1, 7-2,** and **7-3** for sample tests. Allow new employees 30 days to complete the tests, and allow them to tell you when they are ready to complete each portion. Once employees have completed the tests—meeting a predetermined accuracy threshold—they should be expected to comply 100% with the practice's established policies.

Once an oriented employee feels comfortable in the workspace, formal job training can begin. Since few managers have the time to adequately train each person hired, training can become the responsibility of a designated trainer for the practice or the department. There are usually people in a practice who love to teach and excel at it. These people can become your trainers once they have completed trainer's training.

TABLE 7-1. SAMPLE TEST—INFORMATION ABOUT THE PRACTICE

1. How long has the practice been in existence?
2. Who are the physicians in the practice?
3. Draw our organization chart.
4. State our mission and value statement.
5. What is our stated level of service for our patients?
6. Tell me something personal about your supervisor (eg, likes chocolate ice cream, favorite restaurant, children, pets).

TABLE 7-2. SAMPLE TEST—WORKING ENVIRONMENT

1. Where is our supply cabinet?
2. How do we request supplies here?
3. Outline the dress code for your job title.
4. What is our policy for after-hours entry?
5. What is our policy for approval for
   - letters to patients,
   - interoffice memos,
   - e-mail, and
   - web usage?

TABLE 7-3. SAMPLE TEST—HANDBOOK

1. Where are the fire extinguishers?
2. What is the policy for calling in sick?
3. What happens when I need to work overtime?
4. How do I release information on patients?
5. What is the policy on eating in the office?

Ideally, each department will have its own trainer, although in some offices that is not feasible. You may want to designate an administrative work trainer and a clinical work trainer to cover all the job titles and processes in the practice. Regardless of the number of designated trainers, it will be necessary to review what new employees will be shown about their new jobs. As a result, minimum training performance standards should be developed for each job in the office. See **Forms 7-2, 7-3, 7-4, and 7-5** for samples. You will also want to review how each of the performance standards will be presented to the new employee before allowing the trainer to take over the training.

It is vitally important to outline the role of the trainer. Also, the trainer needs to be made aware of the importance of the role in ensuring a new employee's success. Therefore, before assuming their role, trainers must understand that their job is to motivate new employees, tell and show them

FORM 7-2. FRONT DESK RECEPTIONIST MINIMUM TRAINING PERFORMANCE STANDARD

Name of employee: _____

Training Item	Date Reviewed	Date Completed with Approval
❏ Greet patients within 2 seconds of their entering the office suite.		
❏ Use patients' names (Mr/Ms) whenever possible.		
❏ Never call patients by their first names.		
❏ Check patients off the list as they enter.		
❏ Provide new patients with patient demographic form.		
❏ Ask new patients to complete history form.		
❏ Ensure that patients have proper referral authorization.		
❏ Know what to do if a patient does not have proper authorization.		
❏ Enter demographic information into computer.		
❏ Make photocopy of patient's insurance card.		
❏ Make new chart for patient.		
❏ Know what to do when patient is present for appointment and they are not on your schedule.		
❏ Know what to do when the physician is running late.		
❏ Know steps to take when patients ask about their bills.		
❏ Know how to handle an irate patient.		
❏ Know what to do with unruly children in the waiting room.		
❏ Know what to do if you feel threatened by a patient.		
❏ Know how to handle pharmaceutical representatives, vendors, and personal visitors.		
❏ Know special terminology used by the practice.		
❏ Know telephone responsibilities.		
❏ Know how to work copier, fax, telephones, message lighting system, etc.		
❏ Know what to do with records from other providers.		
❏ Know how to handle patients who require special assistance.		
❏ Know how to notify the nurse that a patient is ready.		
❏ Know how to print a superbill.		

how to do their jobs, check that they understand how to do their jobs, observe them doing their jobs correctly, and certify that they have successfully completed their training for the specific tasks.

Trainers should bear in mind that most adults learn by doing. Therefore, for each step in the training program, the trainer should first go over the task and how it is done. The trainer should then demonstrate how to do the task. Finally, the trainer should observe the trainee performing the task successfully.

In order to have new employees retain information, get them involved in the activities. Studies have shown that people retain information when

FORM 7-3. BILLING CLERK MINIMUM TRAINING PERFORMANCE STANDARD

Name of employee: _____

Training Item	Date Reviewed	Date Completed with Approval
❏ Answering telephone, greeting patient by name		
❏ Work flow of practice and how charges are captured		
❏ How diagnosis and procedure codes are assigned in practice		
❏ Policy for changing any code from the one assigned		
❏ Computer training		
❏ Entering charges, diagnoses		
❏ Self-check for accuracy		
❏ Looking up an account balance		
❏ Posting payment		
❏ Review of EOB/write-off		
❏ Self-checking write-off		
❏ Steps to take when payment is denied		
❏ Medicare		
❏ Medicaid		
❏ Private insurer		
❏ Release of information requirements		
❏ Daily balancing		
❏ Where EOBs are filed		

FORM 7-4. NURSE MINIMUM TRAINING PERFORMANCE STANDARD

Name of employee: _____

Training Item	Date Reviewed	Date Completed with Approval
❏ Greet patient		
❏ Use the patient's name (Mr/Ms) whenever possible		
❏ Obtain patient's height, weight, blood pressure, pulse; record in upper right-hand corner of worksheet		
❏ Place patient in a room, and ask patient to change into a gown		
❏ Prepare room for physician's visit		
❏ Place chart in pocket on door and press blue message light		
❏ Locate where injectable meds are kept, and perform log-out processes		
❏ Protocol for giving prescription samples for patient		
❏ How to restock exam rooms each morning, and where each item is placed		
❏ Cleanliness standards for rooms		
❏ Disposal of sharp container that falls		
❏ Ability to perform EKG		
❏ Telephone triage protocols		

FORM 7-5. MEDICAL RECORDS CLERK MINIMUM TRAINING PERFORMANCE STANDARD

Name of employee: _____

Training Item	Date Reviewed	Date Completed with Approval
❑ Flow of patient chart when patient in office		
❑ Flow of patient chart for telephone messages		
❑ How to make up new chart		
❑ Year labels, alphabet labels, patient name		
❑ Order of records in patient chart		
❑ Filing records from other providers		
❑ Standards for keeping charts filed		
❑ Pulling charts for future appointments		
❑ How to handle request for records from other providers in same group		
❑ How to handle request for records from other providers outside group		
❑ How to handle request for records from out-of-town providers		
❑ How to handle request for records from patient's health insurance carrier		
❑ How to handle request for records from disability or auto insurance		
❑ How to handle request for records from life insurance applications		
❑ How to handle request for records from attorneys		
❑ How to handle request for records from other (schools, family members)		
❑ Release information—general		
❑ HIV, AIDS, mental health ailments, alcohol and drugs		

they are emotionally stimulated. What people hear, they forget. What people see, they remember. What people do, they learn. Getting people involved in activities improves morale, stimulates interest, and increases retention.

As new employees demonstrate that they are able to perform each of the functions, the completion date is entered on the training form (**Form 7-6**). Once all the items have been completed, the training record becomes part of the employee's record. The employee is given a certificate to show completion of the training program (**Figure 7-1**).

Training will help employees feel empowered and involved in the organization. When this occurs, they will feel devotion to the organization's purpose. Relationships within the organization will develop naturally. Systems will improve themselves. And the office manager's job will be a little easier.

Once trained does not mean trained forever. Ongoing review and reinforcement will be needed to make sure the employee is performing to standards. Biweekly minichecks should be conducted for the first 90 to 120 days of a person's employment to ensure that information is retained. If lapses are identified, the trainer should reeducate the employee using the same steps as in

FORM 7-6. CERTIFICATION RECORD-KEEPING CARD

CERTIFICATION RECORD-KEEPING CARD

Name: _____   Completion Date: _____
Position: _____   Hire Date: _____

	Certification Components	Tests	Observe	Inspect
1.				
2.				
3.				
4.				
5.				
6.				
7.				
8.				
9.				
10.				
11.				
12.				
13.				
14.				
15.				
16.				
17.				
18.				

Employee Signature: _____

Department Trainer Signature: _____

FIGURE 7-1. CERTIFICATE

Certificate of Achievement   XYZ Medical Practice

This certificate is presented to

Name of Recipient

in recognition of outstanding accomplishments and contributions.

Signature _____   Date _____

Signature _____   Date _____

Organization

the initial training, and note on the training checklist the date of recertification. Recertification can also be updated annually as a review (**Form 7-7**).

What happens if, after training, an individual is still not performing the task correctly? Do you retrain, replace, or modify your expectations? When determining training needs, you will need to assess whether a task is not being accomplished correctly because (1) the employee does not know how to do it, or because (2) the employee knows how but does not do it. The first reason is a training problem and can be resolved with additional training. The second is a management problem and will be not resolved with training.

To determine if the reason a task is not being performed correctly is a training problem or a management problem, ask yourself these questions.

- Has the employee ever done the task correctly?
- Has the employee been taught to do the task correctly?
- If you offered the employee a million dollars right now to do the job correctly, could he or she do it?

If the answer to any of these questions is yes, you have a management issue—not a training issue.

FORM 7-7. YEARLY RECERTIFICATION

YEARLY RECERTIFICATION

Date _____ Areas Recertified _____
_____
_____

Date _____ Areas Recertified _____
_____
_____

Date _____ Areas Recertified _____
_____
_____

Date _____ Areas Recertified _____
_____
_____

Date _____ Areas Recertified _____
_____
_____

Date _____ Areas Recertified _____
_____
_____

Employee Signature: _____

Department Trainer Signature: _____

Bear in mind that training does not create talent. It only refines it. Therefore, money spent to send staff members for training so that they will demonstrate more initiative, more creativity, or a more caring attitude toward patients will in all likelihood be money wasted.

ONGOING TRAINING AND DEVELOPMENT

Although training is usually thought of as initial training for a new job or new responsibilities, training within an organization should be ongoing, formalized, consistent, and valued. Ongoing training and education provides incentive and helps people grow and contribute to the organization's success. However, finding time for that training while you strive to meet the daily challenges of delivering patient care is often difficult.

Coaching on little things frequently will provide consistent reinforcement for the performance standards you have established. **Figure 7-2** shows areas in which to focus mini-coaching sessions. These coaching sessions can be conducted at the general staff meeting, by way of newsletter articles that pertain to the subject, as bulletin board displays, and as topics for the daily lineup.

A daily lineup can be a good way to start the day. The lineup can be an informal meeting in the break room, at the front desk, in the laboratory, or in the manager's office. It focuses attention on one "Basic of the Day" and is addressed by a different person each day. For instance, on Monday the front office supervisor may review the importance of obtaining accurate demographic information and how it is everyone's responsibility to ensure

FIGURE 7-2. MINI-COACHING SESSIONS

Example: Nursing Staff Coaching

Between performance review, coach on...

- Patient relations and hospitality
- Importance of documenting vital signs
- Telephone triage protocols
- Examination room maintenance

- Reporting defects in system
- Submitting ideas for improvements, modifications
- Improving patient care

- Continuous learning and improvement

TABLE 7-4. BASICS OF THE DAY

Day of the Week	Subject	Addressed by
Monday	• Why is obtaining correct patient demographic so important? • What is each person's role in ensuring accuracy?	Front Office Supervisor
Tuesday	• How can we reduce patient waiting time? • Where are the inefficiencies that cause delays?	Nurse Supervisor
Wednesday	• Are we in compliance? • Does the diagnosis in the chart match the one on the claim?	Billing Manager
Thursday	• Telephone etiquette: Is our telephone style helpful, courteous, and professional?	Office Manager
Friday	• Are we working together as a team? • What bumps did we hit this week, and how can we improve?	Office Manager

that the practice has accurate information about patients. **Table 7-4** outlines a sample week's "Basics of the Day". The daily lineup approach to training is an excellent method of directing the organization, focusing attention on matters of importance that affect profitability, enhancing team spirit, and reinforcing professionalism in delivering patient care.

In addition to daily lineups and coaching, ongoing training can be conducted by monthly meetings, newsletters, the Internet, bulletin boards, and lunch-and-learn sessions. You can also provide your staff with books, journals, audio or video teleconferences, and Web-based training.

Among the reasons additional training may be needed are

- changes in regulations, computer systems, or technology require training;
- an employee has taken on additional responsibilities and needs to learn about the new job;
- there is an overall deficiency in an area that additional training may improve (patient relations, communication, teamwork); and
- as a motivator for those individuals who value increased learning and view the additional training as a reward.

MISTAKES TO AVOID

- Not providing good orientation
- Believing we have to do all training ourselves
- Allowing an existing employee to conduct on-the-job training without formalized material
- Believing that the initial training is all that is needed

CHAPTER 8

Evaluating Employee Performance

Jim hated giving employee evaluations. He had been the practice administrator at the clinic for almost 3 years, and he considered this part of the job his darkest hour. He regarded it as time-consuming, emotionally draining, and thankless. The poor performers rarely improved, and those who performed well were disappointed if they were judged less than perfect. However, employee salaries and bonuses were tied to performance evaluations, so they had to be done.

Jim shuffled through the stacks of paper on his desk, jumping from one name to another. In a separate stack were the notes about employee performance he had written to himself throughout the year. He didn't like confrontations, so instead of talking to a staff member about poor performance (or good performance, for that matter), he made notes so that he could address the behavior or give words of encouragement during the annual review. That time was near. He had to have 25 evaluations written by 5 o'clock tomorrow so that he could have them completed by the end of the week. It was going to be a long night.

LESSONS LEARNED

Like Jim, many managers dread employee evaluations. The extra work, emotional involvement, and results make many managers ask, "Why?" And like Jim, many managers make the mistake of waiting to the last minute to complete reviews, and/or they save up a year's criticism to deal with at review time. It is no wonder the review process is a time of emotional turmoil for the evaluator and the person evaluated.

Periodic evaluation and feedback to employees is necessary to keep the wheels of the organization turning smoothly. All employees need to know how they are doing on the job. Some of the most-often asked questions from employees (usually silently to themselves) are:

- How am I doing?
- Am I satisfying my manager?
- How do I compare with others in the same role?
- Is my job performance meeting the expected performance?
- Am I improving?

Many managers fail to communicate the answers to these questions at any other time during the year; therefore, it is no wonder that performance reviews are such an emotional event for both the employee and the supervisor. If the review is tied to monetary rewards, the emotional turmoil is compounded.

The evaluation is a great opportunity for a one-on-one conversation with each staff member who reports to you. It can help you gain new insight into what work is like from that person's perspective; it can provide new ideas; and you may hear suggestions from people who have been thinking about a better way to do things. Therefore, a manager should never do a performance evaluation hurriedly, or treat it as a task that can just be crossed off the list.

Some managers have inherited a performance evaluation program that someone else designed with which they have to live—good or bad. Others have had the privilege (and work involved) of being able to design their own plans. A good evaluation program involves clear, complete, and positive feedback on a regular basis. As the word *program* indicates, evaluation should be more than a once-a-year exercise. This ongoing activity can be broken down into four steps:

1. Here is what is expected of you.
2. Here is what you are doing well.
3. Here is where you need help.
4. Here is what we are going to do about it.

Depending on the size and structure of the practice, the evaluation program can be a comprehensive formalized exercise that the human resources (HR) department uses to determine raises, training needs, promotions and demotions, and termination. Coinciding with these HR functions, the evaluation should have an employee-development component that helps employees reach their full potential and provides them with the feedback and recognition they desire. The evaluation can be instrumental in goal-setting and career development.

Regardless of the size or structure of the organization and the formality or informality of the evaluation, the two main reasons for giving appraisals remain providing feedback to employees on how well they have done and mapping plans for maximum growth and development. The challenge is how you, as a manager, can ensure that these objectives are met.

STEPS IN DEVELOPING A PERFORMANCE APPRAISAL SYSTEM

If you have the luxury of designing a new performance appraisal system from the ground up, you should make sure that all the steps outlined below are followed. If you have inherited an appraisal system, you may need to develop your own internal plan using the steps outlined below to maximize the use of the existing appraisal system.

Step 1: Identify Organizational Objectives

With input from the physicians, directors, other managers, or the planning committee, identify the objectives you want to emphasize. In the medical field, technical accuracy is always of utmost importance. What else do you value as an organization? A review of the mission statement may provide direction in identifying what is important to the organization and what behavior you want to reward. For example, are you looking for innovative people who can find solutions to problems? Do you want employees who make patient care and service to others their top priority? Are you looking for ways to expand and grow, and do you want employees who are dedicated to the growth of the practice? Are basic disciplines valued, such as promptness, a strong work ethic, and unquestionable integrity? Do you value relationship-building so that the practice functions as a family?

This first step may require in-depth analysis to determine exactly where the emphasis will be placed. There may be a need for role-playing to determine which quality is most valued by your organization. You may give examples to the group, such as the following:

Jane is an excellent RN. She has so much knowledge in this field. We know that when she triages a patient telephone call or assists the physician with a procedure, it is done accurately and efficiently. However, Jane has never really had good people skills. She sometimes is abrupt with a patient, and she does not relate well with the other staff members. What is most important—excellent knowledge and technical skill, or good interpersonal relations with the patient?

Once the group has decided on the objectives to emphasize, list those as a starting point for the performance evaluation program.

Step 2: Identify Knowledge and Skills for Each Job	Analyze the jobs being assessed. List each job title, and then list the types of skills and behaviors that are vital to performance of the job. Much of this information can be obtained from the job analysis worksheet you completed in Chapter 4. The staff member who does the billing and claims submission, for instance, needs to know managed care and third-party payer issues and coding, be attentive to details, able to follow through on claims, and should be courteous to patients.

Step 3: Establish Performance Measures	Take the performance measures established in Chapter 7, and list them for each job. When completed, ask the following questions. • Are these standards achievable? • Are these standards understood? • Are these standards as specific and measurable as I can possibly get them? • Are these standards time-oriented? • Are these standards in writing? • Are these standards subject to change?

Step 4: Communicate Expectations	Once the objectives have been identified and the performance measures established, communicate the performance standards to the employees. This should be accomplished before the performance period begins and done with each employee or groups of employees with the same job title. Ask for feedback. It is better to find out now if employees disagree with some of the objectives than during the performance review.

Step 5: Measure Performance	Supervisors need to observe employee performance and results throughout the evaluation period. The person who knows an employee's work best should be the one appraising the performance.

Step 6: Document Performance	Document the performance and results. Documentation ensures that a representative sample of the performance will be used in the appraisal. Discuss the results with the employee in an ongoing manner.

Observation and documentation occur throughout the performance period. As review time nears, evaluate the documentation. Then performance can be measured against desired results.

Step 7: Evaluate and Compile Documented Performance

The next step in the evaluation process is to have another rater evaluate performance. The second evaluator can be a coworker, peer, subordinate, or physician. The added insight into the employee's performance will be valuable in confirming your evaluation or will provide you with new insight into performance.

Step 8: Obtain a Second Evaluation

Guidelines for conducting the performance appraisal are presented in the following section.

Step 9: Discuss the Appraisal with the Employee

After discussing the appraisal, follow up with the employee to reinforce the desired performance and provide guidance where needed.

Step 10: Follow Up with the Employee

GIVING THE PERFORMANCE APPRAISAL

Conducting an appraisal requires skill and tact. A badly conducted session can antagonize and demoralize a good employee, while a well-conducted meeting can be exhilarating and motivating for both the supervisor and the staff member.

The purpose of the performance review is to:

- reach agreement on performance standards,
- identify the employee's strengths,
- identify areas that need improvement,
- reach agreement on career development plans, and
- discuss human resource issues, such as salary increases, promotions, bonuses, and other perks that may be tied to the appraisal process.

Sometimes these objectives are in conflict. Employees hear only that they did not get salary increases or bonuses. Discussion of other job-related areas might have to be postponed until another meeting.

Giving the performance appraisal at an appropriate time will contribute to a successful outcome. Find a time when you and the employee will not be interrupted. The best place is often a neutral private office. It must be a place where the supervisor and the subordinate can be alone, free from interruptions, and without anything separating employee from supervisor. Placing a desk between the supervisor and employee puts the employee at an immediate disadvantage. Instead, try placing the chairs side by side and have coffee and water available. Give the employee advance notice so that he or she understands the yearly review and has adequate preparation time. Open with friendly conversation, discussing sports events, inquiring about family, or commenting on the weather. You need to be comfortable with this. If you have never discussed personal matters, then inquiring about family members is not the right approach.

No one approach is right or wrong. For example, you could list the job strengths first, or use the performance appraisal as a discussion guide. Attaining the objective of the interview may require more than one meeting.

This review is to improve performance, not to comment on personality or lifestyle. One way to avoid evoking defensive behavior from employees is to take an open, nonjudgmental, nonblaming stance. Describing a problem in an impersonal way and encouraging the employee to work with you can help you avoid turning the session into a confrontation.

It is important to bear in mind that regardless of how much care you put into developing a performance appraisal system, the appraisal process does have pitfalls. Common pitfalls include the halo effect, the horn effect, and stereotyping. The *halo effect* applies when a supervisor tends to overrate a favorite employee. This can happen because

- an employee's past record is very good,
- people who are compatible with their managers are sometimes rated more highly than they deserve,
- an individual who does outstanding work immediately before an evaluation may be able to offset an entire year of poor performance,
- a glib talker or a person who has an impressive appearance may be ranked higher than an excellent worker without those attributes,
- a supervisor may be blind to certain defects because he or she also possesses the traits, and
- there is a belief that no news is good news.

Conversely, in the *horn effect,* a supervisor rates an employee lower than circumstances warrant because the supervisor is a perfectionist and expects perfection from all employees. Or perhaps the employee is contrary or a nonconformist, and low ratings are assigned simply because the employee is different. Maybe the person is guilty by association—for example, an individual who is friends with a troublemaker may also be perceived as a troublemaker. Or possibly one bad incident that happened recently offsets an entire year of good work.

Stereotyping involves basing appraisals on fixed conceptions of performance rather than actual performance. It can also occur when standards are subjective and thus have different meanings for different individuals, which confuses the definition of standards and goals.

Sometimes supervisors ignore individual performances and rate all employees the same. Others are lenient and tend to give employees the benefit of the doubt. Consequently, once the performance reviews have been completed, it is important to review, weigh, and judge them to see if halos, horns, or stereotypes have crept into the evaluation process.

Among the benefits that can result from being nonjudgmental are:

- improvement in creativity and problem-solving,
- less supervisory reluctance to discuss employee performance problems,
- clearer understanding by employees of why and how they need to change work behavior, and
- increasing cooperation between individuals.

Turn delivery of the appraisal into an opportunity. Cover one item at a time. Compare the actual results of performance to the standards that have been set. Appraise the employee on accurate and sufficient information. Be honest with the employee, and be prepared to discuss questions. Be open to employee input. Keep written and oral evaluation consistent. Remember that the evaluation is your opinion. Make the written appraisal available to the employee for review. Identify areas for improvement, and support the employee's efforts to improve. Provide a way for the employee to appeal if he or she disagrees with the evaluation. Obtain the employee's signature. And keep everything confidential.

MISTAKES TO AVOID

- Waiting until review time to assess performance
- Basing the appraisal on subjective opinions rather than documented facts
- Conducting the appraisal as a one-way conversation

CHAPTER 9

Retaining Great Employees

Janet, the office manager of a midsized specialty practice, returned from lunch and saw it immediately. On her desk, placed exactly in front of her chair so that she would not miss it, was a white envelope with her name on it. She knew what it was. Many such envelopes had been left on her desk during the past 6 months. She knew it was an employee resignation. She opened the envelope and read:

> *Dear Janet,*
>
> *Please accept this as my notice of resignation. I will be leaving the company effective June 30th, which is 2 weeks from today.*
>
> *Sincerely,*
> *Linda*

Janet was not really surprised. She knew Linda had been unhappy for some time. She had given Linda a raise 3 months before, hoping the money would encourage Linda to remain. It had—for a while. Now Janet looked at the letter and wondered what she could do to stop this revolving door that seemed to be permeating the culture of the organization. It seemed like she was spending most of her time advertising for and interviewing new employees. She was determined that this excessive turnover was going to come to an end.

LESSONS LEARNED

No one can realistically expect to be able to retain every employee. People come and go for a variety of reasons. When people leave jobs, it is rarely because of compensation. More often, they leave because of poor working relationships, lack of respect for senior management, lack of challenge in the work, lack of growth opportunities, or a culture they do not feel comfortable with.

Loss of employees can be very costly to an organization. It is impossible for any organization to build a winning team when it is always playing with rookies. Besides the effect on morale, productivity, and quality of work, the cost of replacing an employee is 150% of the employee's annual salary. There are three types of costs involved:

1. the cost of the person who fills in while the position is vacant, the cost of lost productivity (calculated as a percentage of the base salary), and the cost of severance and benefits;

2. recruitment costs, which involve the cost of advertising, administrative costs, manager's time and pre-employment testing, which can come to as much as 15% of the base salary of the departing employee; and

3. training and new hire costs, which involve administrative costs to put the employee on payroll, establishing computer and telephone hook-ups, the manager's time in building trust and confidence, and the cost of staff training time and tools. These costs are outlined in **Table 9-1.**

At a cost of $75,000 per employee and a 10% turnover rate, turnover expenses can be $750,000 a year. Even on a smaller scale, if the average employee salary is $30,000 per year and there are 20 employees, the cost of turnover for each employee will be $45,000. With a 10% turnover rate—that is, two people per year—the cost would be $90,000.

TABLE 9-1. TRAINING AND NEW HIRE COSTS

Turnover Component	Cost
Cost of hiring replacement (15% of base salary of $50,000/year)	$ 7,500
Training cost (15% of base salary)	$ 7,500
Cost of turnover (85% of base salary)	$ 42,000
Lost productivity cost (35% of base salary)	$ 17,500
Total loss (approximately 150%)	**$ 74,500**

Source: Bliss & Associates, Inc. Available at http://www.blissassociates.com. Used with permission.

WHY EMPLOYEES LEAVE

Most managers and executives agree that hiring and retaining good employees is one of the most important responsibilities a manager has and one with the greatest effect on the organization. Simply wishing for solutions will not produce them; a formalized retention plan supported by the physicians is needed to promote loyalty and reduce turnover. To determine how to encourage people to stay, it is beneficial to first know why employees leave.

Ideally, if you could go back 2, 3, or 4 years and list the positions in your practice and the people who left those positions, you might also be able to trace where they are currently working. Are they working for another physician? Did they move on to a larger organization, such as a hospital system? Or did they change fields completely? You might find that they are still working in the medical field in some capacity. Statistics have shown that people usually remain in the same field. Employees usually do not change fields or occupations—they change employers.

If these people are still working in the medical field, why aren't they still working for you? You can find the answer to that question from an employee survey, through casual conversations, or from exit interviews.

An employee survey provides workers with an opportunity to give honest feedback without revealing their identities. For example, a survey may ask "Do you feel comfortable with the culture of the corporation?" "Do you have a good working relationship with your colleagues?" "On a scale of 1 to 5, with 1 being most important, what are 5 things you would change within the company?" **Form 9-1** is an example of an employee satisfaction survey form.

Another way to find out what employees are thinking is through casual conversations. For example, a manager may want to know how employees view the restructuring of the billing department. Rather than sending out a questionnaire or polling the department staff, the manager may take the opportunity, when she sees a billing department employee getting coffee in the break room, to initiate a casual conversation. After discussing the great coffee aroma and whether the employee's daughter made the basketball team this year, the manager may ask in a friendly way if things are getting back to normal in the billing department. The response may be:

"Oh, they're okay," or "Yes, they're getting back to normal."

She may also hear,

"I don't think they'll ever get back to normal."

A follow-up question from the manager, such as "Why do you say that?" may elicit a response that reveals resentment or morale problems. She may hear, for example,

FORM 9-1. SAMPLE EMPLOYEE SATISFACTION SURVEY FORM

XYZ Medical Practice Employee Satisfaction Survey

Please take a few minutes to complete this survey. Your specific answers will be completely anonymous, but your views, in combination with those of others, are extremely important. To ensure your anonymity, XYZ Medical Practice retained an independent consultant to design the survey, receive the completed questionnaires, and interpret the findings.

1. Overall, how satisfied are you with XYZ Medical Practice as an employer? (Please circle one number)

Very Dissatisfied						Very Satisfied
1	2	3	4	5	6	7

2. XYZ Medical Practice's communication and planning (Please circle one number for each statement.)

	Disagree Strongly				Agree Strongly
I understand the long-term strategy of XYZ Medical Practice.	1	2	3	4	5
I have confidence in the leadership of XYZ Medical Practice.	1	2	3	4	5

3. Your role at XYZ Medical Practice (Please circle one number for each statement.)

	Disagree Strongly				Agree Strongly
I am given enough authority to make decisions I need to make.	1	2	3	4	5
I like the type of work that I do.	1	2	3	4	5

4. Corporate culture (Please circle one number for each statement.)

	Disagree Strongly				Agree Strongly
XYZ Medical Practice's corporate communications are frequent enough.	1	2	3	4	5
I feel I can trust what XYZ Medical Practice tells me.	1	2	3	4	5

5. Your relations with your immediate supervisor (Please circle one number for each statement.)

	Disagree Strongly				Agree Strongly
My supervisor treats me fairly.	1	2	3	4	5
My supervisor asks me for my input to help make decisions.	1	2	3	4	5

6. XYZ Medical Practice's training program (Please circle one number for each statement.)

	Disagree Strongly				Agree Strongly
XYZ Medical Practice provided as much initial training as I needed.	1	2	3	4	5

7. Pay and Benefits (Please circle one number for each statement.)

	Disagree Strongly				Agree Strongly
My salary is fair for my responsibilities.	1	2	3	4	5

Specifically, I'm satisfied with the:

	Disagree Strongly				Agree Strongly
Amount of vacation	1	2	3	4	5

Are there any benefits you would like added to XYZ Medical Practice's benefits package?

Yes ❑   What would you like added? _____

No ❑

8. What can XYZ Medical Practice do to increase your satisfaction as an employee?

_____

_____

_____

"Well, we used to be able to get our work done pretty much by the end of the day. Now, we have papers stacked all over the place, which we can't get to, and the doctors are wondering why their charges are not getting posted. Everyone's getting really tired of the pressure."

Due to this conversation, the manager now has valuable information; that is,

- charges are not getting posted in a timely manner, and physicians are unhappy about it;
- employees are getting tired; and
- employees feel pressured.

Armed with this additional information, the manager may be able to make changes immediately (eg, hiring extra help until work is caught up, offering employees overtime or bonuses to catch up on the work, reviewing the new process to determine what is indeed workable, discussing with the physicians the need to allow the billing department staff to catch up rather than pressuring them to do more).

A well-designed exit interview can also help determine why an employee is leaving and can show what can be done to prevent employees from leaving in the future. The exit interview can be conducted by the manager or a neutral third party to obtain more candid responses from the employee. **Table 9-2** lists examples of questions to ask at an exit interview.

TABLE 9-2. SAMPLE EXIT INTERVIEW QUESTIONS

- Are you leaving this organization to work in another medical practice?

- Are you leaving this organization to work for a hospital or health care organization?

- Are you switching career fields altogether?

- What is your reason for leaving our organization?

- If you could improve only one thing within this organization, what would it be?

- Do you feel that XYZ organization treats its employees fairly and equally?

- Please rank the following criteria in order of importance with 1 being the most important and 5 the least important. What is most important to you in a job?
  _ Salary and benefits
  _ Opportunity for advancement
  _ Friendship with the people I work with
  _ Flexible hours
  _ Driving distance
  Please circle those that you think this organization met successfully

As part of the retention program, you want not only to identify and correct factors that are causing employees to leave, but also to encourage people to stay and be productive contributors. If employees stay only because of pay and benefits, chances are you will not have a good organization. Employees also stay with organizations because of advancement opportunities (the chance to advance their skills or grow toward advancement in a field), job security, pride in their work, openness of an organization, and friendliness and camaraderie of coworkers. Of the five reasons listed, the two influenced least by a manager are advancement and job security. However, the other three—pride in work, camaraderie, and organizational openness—are areas where the manager does have great influence.

Too often, however, managers are dragged down by a myriad of details and lose focus on the real reasons the organization has managers—namely, to motivate employees toward increased productivity and to promote satisfaction among workers. While establishing an employee retention program and administering it successfully does involve a substantial amount of time, it is important for managers to remember that retaining employees will contribute to the profitability of the organization and is far more effective than cutting the cost of office stationary.

DEVELOPING A RETENTION PROGRAM

To develop a successful retention program, it is first necessary to solicit physician involvement. The role of physicians cannot be overstated. They set the style for the medical group's culture and climate.

It is impossible to have good retention unless the physicians recognize the advantages of keeping key employees. Physicians may already be committed to implementing an employee retention program and know the value of keeping loyal and tested workers. If they are not aware of the value of employee retention, they should be made aware of the cost of turnover.

Once you have obtained physician support, you can next look at the responses to the employee satisfaction surveys. These should quickly identify the areas that require your attention. The employee survey and casual conversations in subsequent months will show the progress you've made toward the turnover reduction goal.

An excellent way to increase staff retention is to involve staff members in this process. If they feel involved in the plan and improvements, they will be inclined to remain and work with you in further improving employee retention. This aspect cannot be overstated. Employees prefer good coworkers and a stable work environment. If they know you are interested, they will keep you informed about the progress they observe.

Pride in Work

As discussed, employees stay with an organization partly because of pride in work. Generous helpings of praise and criticism are key ingredients of good staff management, motivation, and retention. Unfortunately, most employees muddle along day after day, without any clue about how they are doing. A few well-chosen, well-timed words from a manager can sometimes do more for an employee's morale than money, promotions, or other tangible rewards. As Mark Twain observed, "I can live for two weeks on a good compliment."[1]

Praise should not be limited to formal performance reviews but should instead be expressed liberally (and sincerely) throughout the entire evaluation period. Following is a list of specific ways to give positive feedback.

- Keep a written record of each employee's good work, such as meeting deadlines and developing good relationships with patients.
- Praise good work publicly when possible.
- At the performance review, ask the employee what he or she has done right since the last review. Allow employees to complete their own review forms, which you'll then examine together.
- Catch staff members doing something right, and commend them for it: "Bob, I noticed you went out of your way to help Mrs Jones resolve her outstanding bill. I just want you to know that I really appreciate your efforts."
- Don't delay giving praise because you feel embarrassed. If too much time passes, the employee may be puzzled when you finally do give praise.
- Don't overdo praise, lest you seem insincere.
- Put the praise in writing. A letter of commendation for the personnel file or a thank-you card can be extremely effective.
- Praise the entire staff as a whole. This establishes a feeling of camaraderie (another reason employees stay with a job).

Giving praise will not just allow you to make an employee feel better; it will also give you important feedback on how to manage the employee in the future. The way a person reacts to praise may reveal clues that can help you manage him or her better. See **Table 9-3** for examples. By noting how staff members respond to praise, you'll have an indication of how to manage them, what to expect from them, and how to address their achievements in the future.

TABLE 9-3. CLUES TO ACTIONS

The Signs	What They Mean
People who respond to praise with disbelief	often try hard to be accepted by those around them, and are willing and eager to please
People who turn praise into a joke	are usually trying to keep a distance from you. They value privacy, wanting to avoid the spotlight
People who pass their share of credit to others	enjoy teamwork and work well with others
People who respond with embarrassment	are usually sensitive, hardworking, and trustworthy
People who react by changing the subject and continuing with the work at hand	are often no-nonsense achievers, independent thinkers, potentially well-organized managers
People who accept praise graciously and easily	are generally assertive, independent, and well-satisfied with their performance and are usually ready to assume more responsibility

Organizational Openness

The second area in which managers can influence employee retention is the openness of the organization. Leaders must work to create a model and atmosphere where change is not feared, but is the norm. This involves promoting and supporting openness to ideas and suggestions, as well as active benchmarking and risk-taking. A key way to encourage the willingness to take risks is to define boundaries for the staff. Let staff members know what mistakes should never be made and in what areas risk-taking and the possibility of failure are acceptable. Openness can also be encouraged by establishing regular meetings where everyone is permitted to express views and opinions about decisions that need to be made, where physicians and staff members interact as peers rather than in a hierarchical relationship, and where new ideas are given a chance to succeed or fail.

How well do you contribute to the openness of the organization? Test yourself. The next time you meet one-on-one with a staff member, tally the number of times you interrupt that person. Also, measure how often you dominate the conversation by noting how many ideas come from you and how often you encourage the staff member to speak and contribute.

In today's workplace, many employees are confronted by rude, inconsiderate, and inappropriate behavior from their colleagues. The third area that influences employee retention is the friendliness and camaraderie of coworkers. To a certain extent, this can be measured before hiring by permitting a new employee to work in the practice for 1 or 2 days to test the waters.

Some 90% of workers responding to a national poll cited instability as a serious problem in the workplace.[2] Instability entails the violation of workplace norms for mutual respect, such as cooperation and motivation. Instability is growing in the workplace, and most people indicate that they want something done about it. In nearly half of the cases of uncivil treatment, the offended worker contemplated changing jobs following the incident.

Coworker Camaraderie

The culture of an organization (ie, what is tolerated, how the leaders behave, what behavior is rewarded) determines the general friendliness and camaraderie of the workplace. It is a manager's responsibility to provide opportunities for friendliness and for relationships to develop on the job. Employees who have the opportunity to get to know each other as individuals (ie, to share food, laughter, and ideas) usually perform better as a team. Developing camaraderie among employees, which includes managers, too, also contributes to a pleasant and productive atmosphere. Among the ways to produce enhanced camaraderie among employees are the following:[3]

- Make your own ice cream or yogurt sundaes.
- Have managers wash employees' cars.
- Sponsor employees in foot races, walkathons, marathons, etc.
- Hold a cookie exchange during the December holidays.
- Bring a bouquet of flowers to work and give it to a staff member with instructions to keep it for 30 minutes or an hour, then pass it on.
- Sponsor summer picnics.
- Have relay races that include who can check a patient in the quickest.
- Hold monthly potluck theme lunches, such as ethnic, western, Polynesian, low-fat, or salad.

Even though some events may cut into work time, the dollar cost to the company is generally small compared to the benefits.

In conclusion, remember that you cannot achieve your goals as a manager if you are continually hiring, training, and working with new employees. The key to your success is to develop a well-trained team that contributes to the overall success of the organization. The only way this can be done is by retaining those good employees you find.

MISTAKES TO AVOID

- Believing that turnover is a fact of life and that nothing can be done to reduce it

- Not considering the cost of turnover when making management decisions
- Not involving physicians and staff members in developing a retention program

Endnotes

1. Prochnow JV, Foulke RA, Prochnow HV Jr. *Toastmasters Treasure Chest.* New York, NY: Harper and Row; 1979.

2. Joyner T. Gen-X: Focus on life outside job fulfillment. *The Atlanta Journal-Constitution,* February 27, 2000:6.

3. Hacker CA. *450 Low Cost No Cost Strategies.* Alpharetta, Ga: Hacker & Associates, 1999.

CHAPTER 10

Bringing Out the Best— Motivating Employees

Downtown Radiology Associates had employed Virginia for several years to transcribe reports for several radiologists. When John, the new office manager, instituted performance objectives for the staff, Ginny fell far behind. John considered terminating Ginny because of her failure to meet productivity standards and the fact that she was often behind in her work. However, when Ginny focused on her job, she was quite good. Her documents looked great, and her error rate was the lowest of all the transcriptionists. So, John looked for ways to motivate Ginny into performing at an acceptable level. He realized while talking with her one day that she had many good ideas about the management of the department. He also learned that she really liked to share those ideas. So John made her an offer. If she met her productivity goals each week, she would not only keep her job, but he would schedule time to listen to her ideas. From that day forward, Ginny's productivity increased dramatically, and John learned that some of her ideas for the department were very useful.

LESSONS LEARNED

A vital part of being a manager is to meet the challenge of motivating employees. Regardless of how good a worker is, how long the worker has been with the firm, or at what level the individual is performing, every employee needs additional motivation from time to time. Commonly, when no motivation is given, the employee moves on to another job. So, like John, not only must a manager determine when to motivate an employee, but the manager must also find the most effective motivator for that individual.

Many times managers know they must motivate, but they make the mistake of trying to motivate all employees with the same rewards. Sometimes raises or bonuses are used as incentives, often with disappointing results. Some managers use perks, such as special parking spaces, employee-of-the-month recognition, or flexible work hours, to motivate employees. Sometimes these perks produce disappointing results. Sometimes, as in the case of John and Virginia, the manager is able to determine exactly what will motivate the individual and achieve success.

DETERMINING APPROPRIATE MOTIVATORS

What is motivation? Charles McConnell describes it as "the initiative or drive causing a person to direct behavior toward satisfaction of some personal need."[1] To provide appropriate motivation for an individual, first determine what needs must be met. There are several ways to do this. One way is to ask employees what they want. This can be done with suggestion boxes, an employee survey such as that discussed in Chapter 9, or talking with them in groups or individually.

Another way to determine needs and appropriate motivators is to use assessment tools, as discussed in Chapter 6. One such tool uses a methodology of action from an individual to indicate how to successfully manage that person.[2] For example, some people enjoy leadership and are motivated by tough assignments and challenges. They will probably respond to the opportunity for growth within the organization. Others tend to be very outgoing, social, and verbally persuasive. They are usually motivated by social recognition, interaction, and situations requiring enthusiasm. Still others look for structure and security, such as job security, a better working space, a financial savings plan, or other long-term benefits. Then there are individuals who love to organize, analyze, and solve complex problems. Motivators for these workers might be awards, rewards, and recognition. Of course, people do not always fit neatly into categories. Outside influences (eg, failing parent, new baby, marital discord, pending move) may determine the factors that motivate an employee.

Another kind of assessment tool is a structure that resembles Maslow's triangle. Maslow's theory is that all human beings have needs, beginning with the most basic (survival) and progressing to more esoteric needs (ie, achievement or self-fulfillment). Maslow's theory is that as basic needs are met, people look for more. Conversely, people cannot really move up to the next level until lower level needs are met. For example, in **Figure 10-1,** individuals would not be concerned about socializing if they were in fear of death. Similarly, motivators on the job will follow the same pattern.

FIGURE 10-1. MASLOW'S TRIANGLE

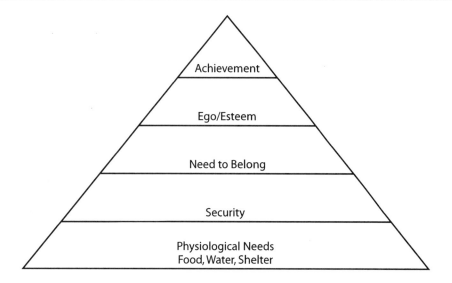

The basic need in working is to earn money to live. Once there is enough to buy groceries and pay for housing, the individual then becomes interested in benefits and security. Health insurance and a 401K plan might be considerations when taking a job. At this point, people begin to be interested in their coworkers. Are they good people to work with? Is it comfortable to work with them? Is it fun to go to work?

The next level is the start of the intangibles. People want to feel important in the organization. Some individuals may want to be in positions of authority where power is vested. Others want to be recognized for the work that they have accomplished, and still others long for ever-increasing goals and challenges.

Being able to recognize where employees are on the triangle and motivating them appropriately is a difficult job for a manager. Although a manager believes a job pays well and offers good benefits and an opportunity for advancement, the employee may view the job differently. Therefore, it is important to recognize indicators of an employee's triangle status in order to gain insight regarding motivation.

As **Table 10-1** demonstrates, the way administrators treat their employees can do more to motivate employees than mere wages. Although money is important to a certain extent, it is not the only motivator (or even the most successful one) in most cases. Take the case of professional athletes. If you told highly paid athletes that you were going to double their salaries tomorrow with only two conditions—that they could not have any fans in the stadium when they played, and that they could not be mentioned on the sports page—how many would accept the proposition? Probably very few, because they have food, shelter, benefits, and security,

TABLE 10-1. EMPLOYEE NEEDS, BEHAVIORS, AND POSSIBLE MOTIVATORS

Need	Identifying Behaviors	Possible Motivators
Physical Needs	• Takes excessive sick leave • Complains of pain, illness • Takes medication, talks about it • Tends to be a loner • Careless about attire and grooming • Generally low work output	• Employee needs professional help before you can motivate him or her
Security Needs	• Worries • Is conservative • Dwells on poor income • Problem with creditors • Talks against company • May have difficulty with eye contact • Procrastinates • May be a loner	• Needs to succeed at something • Credit counseling • Reassurance • Training for advancement
Need to Belong	• Joins civic organizations • Careful about grooming, attire • Easy to get along with • Conformist, goes along with group • Likes to organize events	• Provide social or group contacts • Task force assignments • Buddy to new hires • Provide opportunity to be part of group
Ego	• Displays awards • Name-dropper • Flashy dresser • Does not take criticism well • Will accept challenging opportunities • Takes lead in group • Tends to be impatient • May seek elective office	• Recognize • Provide challenging assignments • Plaques • Trophies • Awards • Letters of commendation • Praise before peers
Achievement	• Fashionable dresser • Can work alone • Patient with others • Feels independent • Requires minimal supervision • Analytical thinker	• Constant flow of challenging assignments and opportunities • Free reign

and they are looking for other motivators—ego and achievement. They want recognition. They want the fans cheering. They want to be reminded that they are at the top of their field.

Motivation can be extrinsic or intrinsic. *Extrinsic factors* involve tangible incentives (money, rewards, bonuses), while *intrinsic factors* are intangible (consistent recognition and praise, for example). Extrinsic factors are usually inducements to comply with organizational requirements. Research suggests that the heavier the use of extrinsic factors to induce behavior change, the more difficult it is to achieve a long-term culture change. Asking for employee input about rewards can give the organization valuable feedback about employee beliefs.

Some ideas for developing intrinsic rewards in a medical practice are recognition, celebration, and culture. Recognition can be public praise, personal notice of appreciation, recognition ceremonies, certificates of achievement, and invitations to meaningful events. Celebration can encompass social events, parties, entertainment, practice anniversaries, seasonal events, and birthdays. Creating a positive and energizing culture can be done by encouraging everyone's participation, asking for opinions and recommendations from individuals, developing internal experts, identifying expected behaviors, eliminating sacred cows, and recognizing all staff as professional in their roles.

Another key factor to consider in determining motivators is the generation of the worker. Recent studies that have focused on motivating factors of younger workers have indicated that such workers like:

- entrepreneurial space and room to fail, rather than micromanagement;
- looking for new ways to do a job;
- training and mentoring, which they consider an investment in their careers;
- a work-life balance, rather than putting in extra time at night and over the weekend;
- clear, concise, and relevant information, such as e-mail;
- fun staff meetings outside the workplace;
- meaningful and challenging work;
- knowing the company's mission and where they fit; and
- community spirit and a place where people care about each other—not a forced team spirit.[3]

Table 10-2 identifies core values and work ethics of different generations of workers and provides insight into their motivators and responses to management.

TABLE 10-2. WORKING GENERATIONS' CORE VALUES AND WORK ETHICS

Type	Number	Defining Events/Trends	Core Values	Generational Personality	Work Ethic
Veterans (1922–1943)	52 million	Patriotism, families, Great Depression, World War II, golden age of radio, silver screen, postwar rise of labor unions	Dedication, sacrifice, hard work, conformity, law and order, respect for authority, hard work before pleasure	Conformers, conservative spenders, absorbed with history and things of the past; believe in logic, not magic	Solid, no nonsense performers with respect for authority and a repository for lore and wisdom
Baby Boomers (1943–1960)	73.2 million	Prosperity, children in the spotlight, television, suburbia, assassinations, Vietnam, Cold War, civil rights movement, women's liberation movement, space race	Optimism, team orientation, personal gratification, health and wellness, personal growth, youth, work, involvement	Driven, soul searchers, willing to go the extra mile, have love-hate relationship with financial prosperity	Tireless movers and shakers and devotees of the corporate mission who are passionately committed to both politics and the spirit of the workplace
Gen Xers (1960–1980)	70.1 million	Watergate, latchkey kids, single parents, MTV, AIDS, computers, Challenger, fall of Berlin Wall, Wall Street frenzy	Diversity, thinking globally, balance, techno-literacy, fun, informality, self-reliance, pragmatism	Self-reliant, risk-takers, skeptical, seek balance and a sense of family, think about the job, not the work hours	Technologically adept, clever, resourceful, independent, anticorporate, comfortable with change, cynical and deeply fragmented
Nexters (1980–)	69.7 million	Computers, school violence, Oklahoma City bombing, TV talk shows, it takes a village, multiculturism, girls movement, McGwire and Sosa	Confidence, civic duty, sociability, morality, diversity, street smarts	Optimistic about the future and realistic about the present, collective action, tenacious	The up and coming "good scouts," willing to work and learn with fresh, easygoing attitudes toward gender stereotyping and traditional expectations

Reprinted with permission from *The Atlanta Journal* and *The Atlanta Constitution.* Joyner T. Generation gaps: workforce at a glance. *The Atlanta Journal-Constitution,* December 19, 1999; P1.

DEVELOPING A REWARDS SYSTEM

There are many things a manager can and should do to motivate employees besides giving cash incentives. The potential to move up within the practice structure can be a great motivator and an incentive to work harder. Promotions can be the ultimate motivator that keeps some workers interested throughout their entire lives. If you use promotion (or the opportunity for promotion) as a motivator, take care to promote those workers who are truly worthy of the promotion. Also realize that a promotion will not be an incentive for every employee.

Some employees will be happier remaining in their current jobs. Ask these people about their likes, dislikes, and job dissatisfaction indicators. Removing one or more of the most unpleasant tasks the employee has may be a reward for that individual.

Other nonmonetary rewards are a mention in the staff newsletter, awards, certificates or trophies indicating outstanding achievement, the opportunity to attend a seminar to learn something new, a party, or a "thank you" or "well done" from the manager or physician.

MISTAKES TO AVOID

- Believing that one kind of motivator will motivate everybody
- Using money to build loyalty
- Failing to understand that recognition and praise can be powerful motivators

Endnotes

1. McConnell CR. *The Effective Healthcare Supervisor.* 3rd ed. Gaithersburg, Md: Aspen Publishers Inc; 1993.

2. *"Disc"* Tool. Scottsdale, Ariz: Target Training International, Ltd; 1996. Target Training International website located at http://www.ttidisc.com.

3. Joyner T. Generation gaps: Work force at a glance. *The Atlanta Journal-Constitution.* December 19, 1999;P1, P6.

Benchmarking, Staffing, and Salary Administration

When consultants reviewed Zenith Multispecialty Clinic's profit-and-loss statement, one of the first items they targeted was personnel cost, which was much too high. The consultants compared the number of fulltime-equivalent employees (FTEs) to industry benchmarking standards and found that Zenith Clinic was substantially overstaffed. The consultants recommended reducing staff numbers by 25%; the physicians agreed; and downsizing began. But after 12 grueling months of low morale, increased turnover, and decreased patient satisfaction, the bottom line did not look any better than it had the year before. The physicians and practice manager decided that it was time to take control of the staffing issues themselves. They resolved to find the right number of staff members for the right amount of money.

LESSONS LEARNED

Expenses related to staff (ie, salary and benefits) make up the major part of all practice overhead expenses, and practices often try to improve the bottom line by cutting personnel costs. Whether you consider the people of the organization the biggest expense or the most valuable asset, the right number of staff members doing the right things can bring greater productivity and profitability to the practice. Conversely, inappropriate staffing (too many or too few employees) can strap the bottom line, deliver a poor product, and become a source of conflict for everyone in the organization.

BENCHMARKING

One way to right-size your organization is to compare it to industry standards, a process known as benchmarking. The productivity and staffing figures of better-performing practices are available from a number of health care management resources. Three resources are:

Practice Support Resources, Inc
2700 Kendallwood Parkway, #104
Gladstone, MO 64119
(816) 455-7790
http://www.practicesupport.com

Cost Survey (annual publication)
Medical Group Management Association
104 Inverness Terrace East
Englewood, CO 80112
(303) 799-1111
(877) 275-6462 (toll-free)
http://www.mgma.com

Healthcare Benchmarks Newsletter of Best Practices (monthly publication)
American Health Consultants
3525 Piedmont Road NE
Building 6, #400
Atlanta, GA 30305
(404) 262-7436
http://www.ahcpub.com

You can access standards for accounts receivable collection, physician productivity, practice capacity, staffing FTEs, and salary, profitability, and operating costs. Used correctly, benchmarking standards can provide a standard for comparison as long as you take into consideration the variances of your individual practice.

Determining Benchmarks

The most important information for which to obtain benchmarks are staffing, physician ratio for comparative practices, and total revenue as it compares to total staff salaries. Then it is necessary to ensure that the standards really apply to your practice and to allow for differences among practices.

How people are used in the practice and what their jobs entail vary from practice to practice, and therefore need to be taken into consideration when you compare your practice to benchmarking figures. For example, staff members with the same job titles may have different responsibilities.

In comparing a receptionist's or patient representative's job responsibilities, it is necessary to determine whether the job entails greeting patients, obtaining demographic information, entering the information into the computer system, and preparing patient charts for physicians. If the job description includes all of these functions, does it also include posting charges, collecting copayments, scheduling appointments, performing telephone triage, and obtaining precertifications and preauthorizations? Similarly, to assess a nurse practitioner's job responsibilities, determine whether that nurse practitioner sees follow-up patients, works after hours in a clinic, takes calls, and sees emergency and walk-in patients; or whether he or she functions more as an RN, assisting the physician with patient care?

Benchmarks also have difficulty in measuring the following factors:

- caregiver resources available to patients between visits. While it may take more telephone and triage time in between visits to manage a patient, these services may result in more efficient care at the time of actual contact.
- payer mix. For example, a fee-for-service visit will add revenue, while a capitated visit will add cost.
- patient's economic status, family support system, insurance coverage, community resources, education level, and occupation. Practices may rely more on nurse triage and walk-in clinics if they are highly capitated.

Benchmarking could also be affected by the practice's demographics. The number and age of the full-time physicians, the number of patients each physician sees, the physician compensation arrangement, and the practice environment influence staff efficiency and productivity levels. Before comparing the organization to the benchmarks, consider the floor plan, the number of examination rooms, the proximity of the nursing stations, and the level of automation in the practice.

Another way to determine the correct staff size is to develop internal benchmarking standards. To do this, compare the number of FTEs to the amount of work performed. Then set realistic goals for improvement, and take steps to move towards those goals.

A common way to determine benchmarks has been to look at staffing ratio by dividing the number of full-time employees by the number of full-time physicians. This comparison does not take into consideration the expectations of the physicians and other environmental and cultural factors. In the ever-changing medical environment, it may be more helpful to compare staffing to RVUs (relative value units) by dividing the total number of RVUs performed over the past year by the number of FTEs. RVUs are the "points" assigned to a medical procedure (CPT™ [current procedural terminology]) codes. Each CPT code is assigned a number of relative units depending on the amount of physician work involved, the practice resources used, and malpractice costs. For example, a level 3 office visit may be assigned an RVU of 1.20, while a hospital admission may carry an RVU of 4.29. Medicare assigns RVUs based on its determination of resources used. Other organizations (eg, McGraw-Hill) use a different RVU base. Regardless of whether a practice uses Medicare or an independent firm's RUVs, the results are the same. The practice can compare units of work performed to the number of people needed to do that work. The resulting in-house benchmark can act as a baseline to determine whether the practice is improving or regressing in its attempt to maximize staff. **Table 11-1** shows an RVU-staffing ratio. Dividing the staff by the RVUs or by patient encounters may show that you are performing better than it appeared when you used straight benchmarking comparisons.

TABLE 11-1. SAMPLE RVU-STAFFING RATIO

CPT Code	Number Performed	Work RVU	Total Work RVUs
99212	1,500	.45	675
99213	2,500	.67	1,675
99214	1,500	1.10	1,650
99215	500	1.77	885
Total RVUs for year			4,885
Divided by FTE			5.00
Total RVU per staff			977

Using Benchmarks

The benchmarking standards of better-performing practices show a total support staff that is larger than the median.[1] The conclusion that can be reached from this is that you should not try to starve a practice into good performance. It is important to remember that the primary objective in benchmarking is to allow the physicians to work at full capacity. In many cases, physician productivity requires adding staff. It is important to make sure that the increased staff has actually had the desired effect.

One of the easiest ways to begin bringing your staffing numbers into line is to ask the following six questions:[2]

1. What do we do now that is a waste of time and could be done more efficiently by someone else?

2. If we were spending our own money, what would we change?

3. What machines, equipment, or technology is available that would do this job better and faster?

4. If I could change my day to get more done, what would I change, and what would be the result?

5. How can we reduce administrative overhead and paperwork?

6. If we could operate in a bare bones environment, what would we concentrate on?

Addressing these questions in the team-working environment will help identify areas for immediate improvement.

It is advisable to determine in advance what improvement you are striving to achieve. Some groups find that keeping the staff-to-physician ratio low helps them achieve balance. Others find that selectively adding staff boosts overall practice productivity. Often, the extra staff members provide clinical support, such as when nurse or a physician assistant is added. Practices rarely raise productivity by adding another layer of administration.

Improvement can be achieved in a number of ways. If productivity is the amount of work divided by the amount of resources, improvement can result from increasing productivity by doing more work with the same resources and holding the quality constant. It can also result from decreasing the input while holding the output constant (productivity remains the same, but staff is reduced). Or improvement can be a result of improving quality while holding input and output constant (doing better with the same or fewer resources).

The principle factors influencing productivity are capital investment, technical change, economies of scale, work methods, knowledge and skill of workers, and the willingness of workers to excel at what they do. While a manager may not have much influence over capital investment, technical change, or economies of scale, managers do influence work methods, procedures and systems, the knowledge and skill of workers, and the willingness of workers to excel. Therefore, if you add staff without showing an increase in productivity or quality, a legitimate question is what you are doing that keeps the staff from being able to keep up with the current demand or workload. Is more staff being less productive? Are you adding staff and adding tasks, too? Are you providing more services, or do you have an untrained staff?

To improve performance, analyze what each staff member is doing. Review job descriptions to ensure each employee is doing the appropriate job. The goal should be to assign each job function to the lowest-paid employee who can perform that function well. For instance, a billing manager with supervisory experience should not be spending a lot of time posting explanations of benefits or making collection calls. Likewise, an office manager should not be doing a billing manager's job. Review what each person is doing during the day and the percentage of time they spend doing it to help determine where you need to realign your staff. There will never be a perfect solution to staffing and equipping a medical practice, but setting goals and striving for improvement can increase the overall productivity and profitability of the practice.

SALARY ADMINISTRATION

How do you keep salaries on track? One of the most useful tools in salary administration is the job description. As discussed in Chapter 4, a job description enumerates the qualifications for a position (education and experience), the responsibilities of the position, and the lines of authority. Before using a job description for salary administration, it is advisable to have the staff member review the description for completeness and accuracy. Once job descriptions have been reviewed, you can develop a salary structure.

Begin by weighing each position. For example, a filing clerk may be Grade 1, a business office manager Grade 6, RNs who are responsible for patient care may be Grade 7, and the practice manager Grade 8.

Once a grade has been established for each job title, determine the baseline wage for each position. The baseline wage is based on supply and demand in your community, so you should do some research to determine the fair market value for each position by subscribing to salary surveys or obtaining information from employment agencies, hospitals, medical societies, and medical management associations.

The next step is to develop a value for the levels of experience. For instance, Level 1 may be a trainee, Level 2 a staff member with 2 or 3 years of experience, Level 3 an employee with 3 to 5 years of experience, and Level 4 someone with 5 or more years of experience. In this example, people with more than 5 years experience would not be paid appreciably more for that experience. There should be a 10% difference between each level, except for the trainee category, for which the difference should be 5%. There should be an average of a 3% increase from the highest level in one grade to the lowest level in the next. **Table 11-2** is an example of salary administration.

The salary administration grid should be reviewed annually to ensure that salaries are still in line with those of other health care facilities in the community. Additionally, if qualified workers are declining job offers because of the pay scale, or if long-term employees are leaving for better paying jobs, steps should be taken to make the pay scale competitive.

The bottom line is that the staff and ancillary services must provide patients and physicians with efficient service. This builds practice revenues by keeping patients satisfied and making the most of every group's most valuable resource—its physicians' time.

TABLE 11-2. SAMPLE SALARY ADMINISTRATION GRID

Position	Level	Experience	Salary	Explanation
Grade I— File Clerk	1 2 3	Trainee 1 year 2+ years	$18,000 x $18,900 (x + 5%) $20,790 (x +10%)	
Grade II— Front Desk Patient Service Representative; Nurse Techs; Collector	1 2 3 4	Trainee 1-2 2-3 3+	Add 3% x x + 5% x + 10% x + 10%	
Grade III— Charge and Payment Poster	1 2 3 4	Trainee 2-3 3-5 5+	Add 3% x x + 5% x + 10% x + 10%	
Grade IV— Nurse	1 2 3 4	Under 2 2-4 4-7 7+	Add 3% x x + 5% x + 10% x + 10%	
Grade V— Billing Office Supervisor	1 2 3 4	3-5 5-7 7-10 10+	Add 3% x x + 5% x + 10% x + 10%	
Grade VI— Nursing Supervisor	1 2 3 4	4-5 5-7 7-10 10+	Add 3% x x + 5% x + 10% x + 10%	
Grade VII— Practice Manager	1 2 3 4	3-5 5-7 7-10 10+	Add 3% x x + 5% x + 10% x + 10%	

MISTAKES TO AVOID

- Cutting staff to save money without performing a productivity analysis
- Not establishing internal benchmarks
- Adding staff without improving quality or productivity

Endnotes

1. Larkin H. Groups get the most from staff and ancillary services. *MGM Update.* March 1, 1999.

2. Fogel PA. Benchmarking and action. *Healthcare Financial Management Magazine.* July 22, 1999.

CHAPTER 12

Conflict Resolution

Tony, the practice manager of Downtown Clinic, and Frances, the central billing office manager, met on Thursday afternoon to discuss critical issues. Tony and the practice's physicians were not happy with the current system because it seemed that no matter how hard they worked, their revenues didn't increase. They were unhappy with performance reports they received and the amount of money being collected. Frances and her staff were equally as frustrated. With a highly profitable practice producing high gross charges and an acceptable collection rate, billing office staff members believed that they were doing a good job. However, they were having difficulty getting correct information from the front office. Often, claims were rejected because a patient's name or insurance information was entered incorrectly. When they raised these issues, they were told, "It is a billing office problem." The executive committee and Frances met to resolve these issues. After discussing the situation for more than 2 hours, both sides walked away without reaching a satisfactory conclusion. Tony and Frances knew that this problem would require more of their time in the future.

LESSONS LEARNED

Managers spend approximately 20% of their time resolving conflicts ranging from whether to change billing services and how to assist physicians and nurses to determining who took the last bagel out of the refrigerator. Conflict—tension that exists when parties have competing goals—has four major sources:

1. Competition for limited resources. Conflict can result if an individual sees that someone else's success diminishes the chances of his or her own success.

2. Clashes of values. Conflict can result because of differences in work values or personal or cultural values.

3. Poorly defined responsibilities. Conflicts can arise over who is in charge of what portion of the office and/or of the way things are done.

4. Change. Whenever there is change, there will also be resistance to that change.

Conflict is not bad in itself. Depending on how it is managed, it can have productive or destructive results. When conflict diverts energy from important paths, decreases productivity, destroys morale, polarizes the group, and builds distrust, it can have a devastating effect on an organization. However, it can also open issues to discussion, promote a solution to a problem, and lead to greater understanding between the individuals or groups. Rather than being viewed as a problem, conflict can be viewed as an indication that something needs to be changed.

Many people associate conflict with anger, fear, anxiety, or frustration and believe that the only way to deal with it is to eliminate the source of the conflict. Americans tend to resolve disputes by fighting, voting, litigating, or appealing to authority. These methods share two characteristics: someone must lose, and everyone must accept the process and agree to its outcome.

Alternative processes, such as negotiation and mediation, require thinking strategically to persuade people and foster cooperation. Successful managers use negotiation and mediation in conflict resolution. In arbitration, the involved parties are bound by law to accept the decision of the arbitrator. Arbitration is often used in labor union disputes. Mediation, on the other hand, is more of a handshake agreement that both parties accept.

CONFLICT DIAGNOSIS

As a manager, you may be a participant who is emotionally involved in the conflict, or you may be a mediator or negotiator. To help you reach the best resolution in either case, use the following model as an aid in judging the difficulty of reaching a satisfactory outcome.[1] (See **Table 12-1.**) The model consists of seven dimensions of conflict and shows the difficulty of reaching a satisfactory outcome for each dimension. The more of the dimensions that are easier to resolve, the easier it is to reach a resolution for the conflict as a whole.

TABLE 12-1. CONFLICT DIAGNOSTIC MODEL

Dimension	Difficult to Resolve	Easier to Resolve
1. Issue in question	A matter of principle	Can be broken down into smaller issues
2. Size of stakes	Large	Small
3. Interdependence of the parties	Not acknowledged	Positive
4. Continuity of interaction	Single event	Long-term relationship
5. Structure of the parties	Divided, with weak leadership	Cohesive, with strong leadership
6. Involvement of third parties	No neutral third party parties	Trusted, credible, and neutral third party available
7. Perceived roles in conflict	Unbalanced: one party feeling more harmed	Parties perceive harm equally

The involvement of a trusted, credible, and neutral third party often makes conflict easier to resolve. As a manager, you are often called on to act as that neutral third party. It is vitally important to be viewed as trusted, credible, and neutral in order to help bring about an end to the conflict and come up with a solution acceptable to all involved parties. The responsibilities of the third party are to gather information about the nature and scope of the problem and mediate an agreed-upon solution. **Table 12-2** outlines the steps in conflict management and presents poor and better ways to conduct the session.

It is important to bear in mind that not every attempt is going to work. An agreement may not be reached at this particular time, but the disputants may agree on a smaller issue.

It is also important to remember that the agreement that the disputants reach may not be the agreement that the mediator sees as fairest or best. For instance, if the disputants compromise, it may not be a 50-50 compromise. When this happens, it is best for the mediator to stay out of the resolution as long as the compromise is mutually agreeable to both parties.

If a disputant makes an extreme suggestion for resolving the conflict, such as, "Why don't you just fire her?" the mediator should accept the suggestion without comment and take it to the other disputant—"Bill believes that the best way to solve this is to fire you." The other person can then respond to the suggestion. The goal is to help the disputants develop

TABLE 12-2. CONFLICT RESOLUTION

Step	Principle	Poor	Better
1.	Interview disputants	One at a time	All together
2.	Maintain control	Get off topic	Remain focused
		Bring up issues from the past	Remain focused on current issue
		Allow outbursts in order to be the nice guy	Stop outbursts and rudeness immediately
		Assert control forcefully	Control indirectly
		Have disputants sit across from each other	Have disputants sit in chairs all facing you (put angriest disputant in softest chair)
		Allow disputants to talk to each other	Have disputants talk only to you. Use phrase "talk to me."
3.	Establish rapport	Deciding who is right	Understand each disputant's story as he/she sees it
4.	Don't agree or sympathize	Reassure, console	Remain distanced
		Allow yourself to be drawn in by answering questions	Ignore disputant's questions
5.	Talk too much	Do most of talking	Disputant's talk 80% of time
6.	Don't allow yourself to be interviewed	Answering disputant's questions, such as "why does she act that way?"	Ignore disputants questions
7.	Don't lead disputants	Second-guess disputants	Find out how each disputant sees problem
		Ask questions that lead to an answer you have in mind	Keep questions neutral
8.	Avoid closed questions	Can be answered with a single yes or no	Ask questions that require disputant input
9.	Keep on the topic	Allow disputants to tell other people's views	Allow disputants to tell only their points of view
		Ramble into unrelated problems	Keep disputants talking only to you
10.	Mediate only one problem at a time	Allow a backlog of problems to surface	Focus on one particular problem
11.	Get specific information	Allowing inferences to be discussed, such as "Alice is inconsiderate"	Keep focused on actions, such as "Alice went into the cafeteria and didn't ask if I wanted anything"
12.	Avoid making suggestions	Mediator resolves issue by making suggestions	Disputants resolve conflict by working it out themselves

a mutually agreeable action plan. Even if the resolution does not seem fair to you, you have increased the chances that both parties will adhere to the compromise and consider the matter resolved.

As a manager in a highly stressful field, it is very likely that you will be drawn into conflicts with staff members, physicians, other departments in your organization, vendors, and outside organizations. In dealing with conflicts, bear in mind that there are three basic management conflict styles:

- cooperation,
- competition, and
- avoidance.

Table 12-3 indicates the differences in the characteristics of these conflict management styles.

TABLE 12-3. CONFLICT MANAGEMENT STYLES

Cooperation	<ul><li>Motivated to understand opposing views and needs</li><li>Understands shortcomings in own perspective</li><li>Looks for other ideas, needs</li><li>Strengthens relationships</li><li>Considers problem a mutual one</li></ul>
Competition	<ul><li>Vigorously defends his or her own position</li><li>Prefers to find weakness in opposing arguments</li><li>Focuses on undercutting other positions</li><li>Resorts to using authority or power to impose solutions</li><li>Wants to win at the expense of others</li></ul>
Avoidance	<ul><li>Is often unaware that anyone else is experiencing conflict</li><li>Assumes that others agree</li><li>Sees little need to explore others' opinions</li></ul>

Adapted from American Society for Training and Development. *Coming to Agreement: How to Resolve Conflict.* INFO-LINE #8909. Sept 1989.

Conflict management is a skill; it can be learned. Once you have identified your own conflict management style, you are better able to handle the conflicts that come into your own professional life. When dealing with professional conflicts, use the following principles of conflict resolution.

- Understand that even though positions seem incompatible, you do have compatible interests, and your goal is to reach those interests.
- Every side usually has something valuable to say.
- Developing a dialogue will allow parties an avenue to resolve their conflicts.

- There are areas where parties agree. It is important to start with those areas.
- Using a relaxed, confident tone when discussing conflicts will promote resolution.
- State your needs only after contact and good will have been established with the other parties.
- Both parties cannot state their needs at the same time.
- Sometimes listening to the other party's needs will be more effective in getting you what you need.
- To promote effective communications, give the other person your time and attention.
- Clarify what was being said through questions and paraphrasing. For instance, "Do you mean that . . . ?," or "In other words, you feel that . . . ?"
- After repeating and rephrasing the other person's statements, build on them.
- Pull from what is communicated through body language or avoidance of important issues.
- Provide occasional affirmative responses, such as "Uh-huh" or "I see."
- Search for the cause of the conflict, not for placing blame.
- After both parties have stated their needs, restate what is important to you and what you perceive is important to the other party.
- Seek closure at the end of the discussion by summarizing the points made and agreed to.
- If you find that you cannot resolve the conflict by using these methods, then it may be time to find a third party to whom you and the other party can vent, so that a resolution can proceed.

In all conflicts, bear in mind that the cause of the dispute often is misperception, and that the dispute indicates a need for change. This can be an excellent opportunity to clarify expectations, build cohesiveness, and create a problem-solving atmosphere.

MISTAKES TO AVOID

- Not addressing conflict as it develops
- Trying to find remedies for other parties rather than allowing them to work it out
- Allowing yourself to be drawn into other's conflicts

Endnote
1. Greenhalgh L. *Sloan Management Review.* Summer 1986.

CHAPTER 13

Managing Change

Eleanor had been manager of the billing office for Specialty Care Associates for almost 5 years. Things were not going as well as the physicians expected them to. Because of several new managed care contracts, a transition of staff in the office, and the heavy workload, the receivables had declined for more than 3 months in a row. Eleanor thought that if she assigned the billing staff to teams to work on accounts together, rather than continuing with the production-line method, things would improve. However, staff members had experienced several changes over the past 6 months, and she was reluctant to force yet another change on them. So, she gathered them together and said,

Here's the problem. I have doctors over here who want to be paid. I have managed care companies over there that owe us money. Somehow, we need to get that money over there in here better and faster so that everyone can be paid.

There was some general complaining from the staff members, a little finger-pointing, and some grumbling before Eleanor continued:

I've explained the problem. I'm not going to tell you how to solve it, but I do want you to come up with a solution.

Eleanor then left the staff members alone. She noticed that they had a rather lengthy meeting with lots of energized discussion before going home for the day, and that one person seemed to have taken charge of the project.

Eleanor hoped she had done the right thing by turning the problem over to the staff. She crossed her fingers and waited. Several days and many meetings later, the staff members came to her with an idea about how things could work better. The spokesperson explained that many times they found themselves duplicating work because one person had worked on posting a check to an account and started the review process, and then the collections person received the account and started the review process over again. They thought it would work better if they divided into teams rather than work as a production line.

Eleanor agreed, and the team concept was put into action. Although there were a few employees who did not accept the change, most staff members had been involved in the decision and wanted it to work.

LESSONS LEARNED

Change is rarely greeted with cheers and applause, whether it is a result of new leadership, a merger, the acquisition of a practice, an internal reengineering effort, or simply the introduction of a new patient demographic form. Generally speaking, we are creatures of habit who create comfort zones and routines. We usually arrive at work at the same time each day, grab a cup of coffee, greet the same people as yesterday, and perform our jobs with routines we have established. A misplaced stapler, a different chair, an unscheduled meeting, or a crisis that erupted before we arrived at the office can throw us out of kilter for the entire day. It should be no surprise that major changes such as computer upgrades, change in patient flow, mergers, acquisitions and reengineering can result in operational chaos, general wailing, and staff turnover.

Nonetheless, change is a reality of organizational life. It is necessary to achieve growth, promote economies of scale, and establish referral sources. Poorly managed change can result in lowered organizational commitment and satisfaction. It can promote behaviors that work against what the organization is attempting to accomplish.

As a leader, you are faced with change when you want to revise operations or when the physicians or executive committee make decisions for change and assign you to implement it. Occasionally, you may be faced with something completely beyond your control, such as being acquired by another entity or merging with another practice.

The way you view the change and the message you send to your staff will directly affect the chance of a successful outcome. If you feel threatened by the impending change, you may have a difficult time conveying a positive message to the staff. It is of vital importance to manage yourself first. A better understanding of the dynamics involved in change and a little self-analysis may enable you to bring about a successful transition.

The self-analysis tool in **Form 13-1** is designed to provide insight into your own change acceptance quotient (CAQ). For this assessment, assume that you are office manager of a midsized practice and have just been informed that the physicians have decided to merge with another group. The change is scheduled to take place within the next 6 months. On a scale of 0 to 10, rate your reaction to this decision. Once rated, add up your answers to arrive at your CAQ. Now, go back and consider these same questions, as if the merger will not happen until sometime next year. What is your CAQ now? Next, assume that you have just come up with a better way to conduct the patient intake process, and you want to make a change. What is your CAQ under these conditions?

You probably saw a difference in your acceptance of change depending on whether it was your idea or whether the change was thrust on you. So it should come as no surprise that you must involve the parties the change will affect. This is true whether you are trying to change the patient intake process, hire a new physician, or merge with another organization. Employee motivation and performance improve dramatically when employees have a stake in the organizational results.

FORM 13-1. SELF-ANALYSIS TOOL

How do you view change?

1. Threat	0	2	4	6	8	10	Opportunity
2. Holding on to past	0	2	4	6	8	10	Reaching for future
3. Immobilized	0	2	4	6	8	10	Activated
4. Rigid	0	2	4	6	8	10	Versatile
5. A loss	0	2	4	6	8	10	A gain
6. Victim of change	0	2	4	6	8	10	Agent of change
7. Reactive	0	2	4	6	8	10	Proactive
8. Focused on past	0	2	4	6	8	10	Focused on future
9. Separate from change	0	2	4	6	8	10	Involved in change
10. Confused	0	2	4	6	8	10	Clear

What is your CAQ?

CAQ	Rating
0-20	Poor. Not a recommended change leader. Should seek professional help in accepting change.
20-40	Below Average. Suggest working on accepting change by varying daily routine.
40-60	Average. Definitely not a change leader, however, will probably accept change once it is implemented.
60-80	Above average acceptance of change. Good candidate for change leadership.
80-100	Outstanding acceptance of change. Probably goes out of way to do things differently.

Adapted from American Society for Training and Development. *Coming to Agreement: How to Resolve Conflict.* INFO-LINE #8909. Sept 1989

There was probably also a difference in your CAQ when the change was an internal one (creation of a new internal process) as opposed to an external one (merger with an outside organization), and when change was imminent in contrast to when there was time to grow accustomed to it. Generally, slow change is easier to accept than quick change, and internal changes are more readily embraced than external changes. **Table 13-1** suggests the degree of difficulty in implementing a change based on these key indicators.

TABLE 13-1. DEGREE OF DIFFICULTY IN IMPLEMENTING CHANGE BASED ON KEY INDICATORS

Easier to Manage	Internal Input Slow	Internal Input Fast	Internal No Input Slow	Internal No Input Fast	External Input Slow	External Input Fast	External No Input Slow	External No Input Fast	More Difficult to Manage

Adapted from *Journal of Medical Practice Management.* 1998; 14:23-27.

IMPLEMENTING CHANGE

To orchestrate any change, it is important to understand the three basic phases of change. Phase 1, the formative phase, is the time the concept of change comes into being. There is a search for something new, and a strong sense of mission prevails. There is also a lot of tension and uncertainty during this phase, with questions such as "Are we doing the right thing?," "Is this really going to work?," and "Why can't the rest of them see what a great concept this is?" This is the phase where things happen.

In Phase 2, the normative phase, the organization has come through the tunnel and is back in the light. The fine-tuning process begins. There is increased structure as people learn their new roles and stability replaces the high energy level of Phase 1.

In Phase 3, the integrative phase, the organization takes on a new direction, and a new culture emerges.

Phase 1: Formative

For the most part, change is beyond control of the line staff, so it is important to consider what effect the change will have on them. Their actions and behaviors will be key to successful implementation of the change.

Some employees will be angry about the change and may either hold in their anger, allowing it to fester, or spread their unhappiness to other employees. Some employees will feel a lack of direction. They may scurry around trying to look busy but will not be accomplishing anything. Others will try to hold on to what was rather than to look at how things will be. They may be given new job assignments or new ways of doing their jobs, but they revert to the old ways of doing things. Some employees will quit—and go. Others will quit—and stay. Still others will adopt an "ain't it awful" attitude and align themselves with others of the same opinion.

Because of the potential effect of these reactions, people issues cannot be ignored. The manager's role is to minimize the negative reactions and promote acceptance of the change. Regardless of how good the reason for change, it will still cost someone something and bring someone's familiar world to an end. If you can determine ahead of time where the greatest effect will be, you can plan to help those individuals during crucial times.

You also need to assess the readiness of the organization to accept change. Although change is always unnerving, some organizations are better equipped to cope with transition than others. The culture of the organization will affect the openness to change. If trust has been established and there is open communication and a team spirit, change will be less disruptive than if morale is low and discontent and suspiciousness are present.

Every change also has political implications. Being able to analyze the political climate and forecast trends will help you avoid problems during the transition phase. For example, in many mergers and acquisitions, there is a change of power. Supervisors who once had fifteen people reporting to them, now find they have no one. Managers who had a great deal of control over their work environment may now find that their former power, control, or authority has been greatly diminished or disappeared completely. Often, people are jockeying for positions of leadership, and no one is certain who will be the winner. This uncertainty causes stress not only for the individuals involved directly in the change of power, but also for their subordinates.

If the leaders can work out details ahead of time of who will be in charge and what the organization chart will look like, they can relay that information to the organization's members. If the members know what to expect, have confidence that someone is in control, and perceive structure rather than anarchy, the change will come about with few casualties.

Many organizations find that the creation of a transition team will help obtain buy-in from people at all levels of the organization. Get input from a cross-functional team of individuals. Select key individuals for the team. For example, if you are looking at revising billing and reimbursement processes, a biller, a patient account representative, a front desk staff member, and a volunteer should be participants.

Use a flip chart and colored markers to chart out the key processes as they are operating currently, and then discuss how steps can be eliminated and how technology can shorten those process times. Retool the forms that are used, and look at job descriptions to make sure that they are still applicable to the new process. Construct a comprehensive implementation time line with dates and interim deadlines. Set goals for measuring the improvements. Communicate all changes to the staff long before making them. Hold regular meetings to determine which systems work smoothly and which need additional fine-tuning.

Ensure that the physicians are in sync with what you are trying to accomplish. The speed at which the new culture is established and increased productivity is realized depends on the physicians' leadership and commitment to change.

During the implementation period, provide proactive troubleshooting. This can include writing and distributing weekly updates, listening to staff members when they say something may not work and asking them to find another solution, and using e-mail or another fast way to get the word out quickly to as many people as possible.

Phase 2: Normative

The second phase—the attempt to return to normality—may be much like opening a new office or rebuilding from the ground up, or it may be very low key. Probably the most overlooked feature of the change process is staff training. Just because new protocols and job descriptions are in writing does not mean that staff members fully understand their new roles. Comprehensive training is critical to the success of any change. For example, in addition to providing training on a new computer system, it is advisable to offer an intensive overview of new protocols and job descriptions and to start out on the right foot by setting up some dry runs of the new procedures.

Rewards are also important. The emotional toll on employees should not go unnoticed. Group pizza parties or picnics, gift certificates to movies or video stores, or sporting events may jell the group into the new culture you are seeking.

Phase 3: Integrative

When mergers and acquisitions take place, a new postmerger culture is inevitable. This is no less true with reengineering and restructuring a practice. Any change in the practice will bring a change in its culture.

There are ways to control the change in the culture. Make sure to discuss values, vision, and heritage when negotiating a merger or reengineering. Design structure and systems to reflect the new organization's vision. Create a sense of urgency for the new culture.

Merge and redesign operational and clinical systems. Translate values into behaviors, and measure whether those behaviors are occurring. Serve as a role model for the new culture. And create incentives that promote the new culture and measure whether the culture is shifting.

Although most people responsible for initiating change realize that it will take time before things are back on an even keel and the new culture has begun to take effect, the fallout from the change usually takes 3 to 6 months longer than was originally anticipated. In some instances, creating a postmerger culture has taken as long as 10 years, and sometimes the new entity is unsuccessful in creating a cohesive new culture. To make the change less painful:

- Ensure all physicians are fully committed. Physicians who are not can be destructive to the process.
- Clearly define your change vision. What will this new organizational process look like when it is finished? Are the steps written down on paper? Are processes or changes graphed and charted so that staff members and physicians can visualize them?
- Set objectives for where you want to be in 90 days, 6 months, and 1 year.
- Ensure you have nonphysician leaders who understand the goal and can empower and lead the staff members through the process.
- Hold regular staff meetings to determine what worked, what did not work, and how things can be improved.
- Assign a physician manager to each area that is being reengineered.
- Budget for change. Staff members are going to incur overtime, and new equipment will need to be purchased, so prepare in advance for these expenses.
- Train. Train. Train. No amount of training will ever be overtraining.

MISTAKES TO AVOID

- Underestimating the toll that change will take
- Overlooking staff members' feelings and concerns
- Making changes quickly without involving people